"I've had to paste on fake wrinkles for half the parts I've played: Henry VIII, Andrew Jackson, Cardinal Richelieu, Thomas Jefferson; but you can peel those off at the end of the day's shooting. This book looks like a good way to avoid real wrinkles. It is is a valuable guide to a healthy life."

Charlton Heston
Actor

◇

"I love this book. It opened my eyes to some new and healthy avenues for living."

Chad Everett
Actor

◇

An invaluable book of information and reference on health care. This book tells you what to expect and what to do about it."

Ann Jeffreys
Actress

This book is dedicated to
Lori, Judi, and Shari,
my three health-minded daughters.

Rejuvenate

Devra Z. Hill

AVERY PUBLISHING GROUP INC.
Garden City Park, New York

The health information and opinions contained in this book are based upon the training, personal experiences, and research of the author. Because each person and situation is unique, the author and publisher urge the reader to check with a qualified health professional before using any product or procedure where there is any question as to its appropriateness.

Because there is always some risk involved, the author and the publisher are not responsible for any adverse effects or consequences resulting from the use of any of the suggestions in this book. Please do not use the book if you are unwilling to assume such risk. Feel free to consult a physician or other qualified health professional. It is a sign of wisdom, not cowardice, to seek a second or third opion.

CONTENTS

CHAPTER 1
The Air and Mental Attitude Affect Our Faces

Wrinkles used to come with old age but today I see young people in their twenties starting to wrinkle and age before their time.

I don't know anyone who wants to look old and really nobody has to if they put forth a bit of effort. Since I have researched this problem I know there are ways to prevent premature aging and even ways to delay the signs of time passing when they usually begin to appear.

Most of us know that certain diets and exercises can help us stay healthy and youthful, but there is a little more to it than what is generally known. I have found a 5 point plan that works wonders for me and my friends. Basically it encompasses:

1. The air and mental attitude
2. Diet, supplements, and acid/alkaline balance

3. Body and facial exercises and sleep
4. Colonics and/or enemas if needed
5. Really knowing yourself

To some this will sound familiar, to others it may sound completely foreign or even ridiculous but to anyone interested in looking and feeling great it will be of tremendous help.

In our half of the 20th Century we are all living in future shock.This means with over-population, pollution and inflation our lives are filled with the type of stress that ages us fast.

I have seen myself and some of my friends go through a particularly stressful situation and literally age overnight. Stress in life is unavoidable and aging is the bad effect of stress. But some stress is good. That would be stress caused by competition in exercise, business or a creative outlet. That kind of stress stimulates us to be better. But the stress of emotional and mental problems plus pollution and inflation added to over-crowding has a very depressing effect on everyone. However, it is possible to rejuvenate ourselves.

I consider old age a burdensome disease but at this point in time it is an epidemic and everybody gets it eventually. Hopefully in the near future science will find a way for us to look good till we die and with a bit of luck and a lot of intensive research we may even avoid that depressing end. However, right now the longer we can delay looking old the better we will feel.

That is the reason for this book. I will condense 8 years of study into these pages because I want to share my "Looking and Feeling Great" secrets with you. I believe if you feel better, I'll feel better. This is a simple truth. In general we seem to be living in a negative world and negative feelings are transferred from one person to another. I believe many people are negative because they just don't feel good and that causes them to look bad. Often we don't seem to know what is wrong with us but we have a vague feeling of the "blahs." The blahs usually start with the polluted air we breathe. Most of the time we are not getting good clean oxygen and our bodies know it even when we don't. Clean air is vital to total physical and mental health and there is no doubt that it makes us look better. It brings a sparkle to our eyes and a bloom to our cheeks, giving us a glow.

Metropolitan areas have really become a problem but even the air in our rural areas is not clean anymore. We not only have smog from industry and transportation but we have fallout from the nuclear industry and spraying contamination from pesticides and other chemicals. A dental technician I know wears a little shield on her lapel that tells when she has had too much radiation from working around x-ray machines. She had not taken any x-rays in three days but she did walk outside the metropolitan Los Angeles area and after a few days her shield registered danger. So it is easy to see that pollution is everywhere. Pollution decreases oxygen and oxygen is the blueprint of all life. And believe it or not, pollution makes us frown. When we frown or look tense and unhappy we pull down about 60 facial muscles and we certainly don't need to help gravity pulls us down. However, when we laugh we pull up about 13 facial muscles, plus spontaneous laughter increases blood circulation and this in turn nourishes the face and reduces wrinkling.

Another major problem with our air today is one that most people know nothing about and that is that pollution causes too many positive ions in the air throwing off the balance between positive and negative ions. An ion is an atom or molecule with an abnormal number of electrons. When an external force knocks an electron out of the orbit of a normal, uncharged atom or molecule, it becomes a positively charged ion; and when that freed electron attaches itself to another atom or molecule, a negatively charged ion is created. The molecules of oxygen that we breathe and the hydrogen with which it combines to form water have been ionized in this way. They are acted upon by ultra-violet rays and other radiations from the sun and space, by emissions from radioactive substances near the surface of the earth and air turbulence or friction.

Negative ions are called "Vitamins of the Air" by many in the health field because they restore the air's natural freshness. Negative ions are found in abundance near beaches, waterfalls, forests and high in the mountains. That's one of the reasons people go to these areas for fun and relaxation.

Unfortunately, most of us live in asphalt jungles and spend much of our time inside houses, stores, apartments or factories. We do not receive enough sun and fresh air and as a result we become agitated, anxious or drowsy, short of breath, stuffy and sometimes experience aches in our joints or muscles. Very few of us attribute this to a lack of negative ions. Negative ions move in a zigzag pattern in the air and transmit their negative charge to bacteria, dust, smoke particules and water droplets. The negative electrical charge gathers these particles together and drops them to the ground keeping them from getting into our lungs. An adult circulates about 2,500 gallons of air through the lungs in 24 hours. This amounts to about 15 thousand million ions. So now how do we get more healthful negative ions? Well, we either decide to move to better air or we decide to do something about the air where we are presently living. You can live without food for 60 days, without water for 7 days, but without oxygen you won't make it past 2 minutes.

If you don't want to take the time to write to your representative and complain about air pollution, and believe me they do listen to what their constituents say, then you can buy a negative ion machine at many of the health food stores and put it in the room where you spend the most time. Often these machines are advertised in health magazines. Also ferns give out negative ions. They do help somewhat and a little help is better than none at all. But, of course, the best help would come from cleaning up our environment. The excuse we get from big business and government is that pollution comes with progress. Well, we are paying dearly for our progress in the price of excess pollution which accelerates our aging process and our wrinkles to say nothing of the fact that it is literally killing us.

One of the most important ways to slow down the aging process with the air we breathe is not to smoke. Practically everyone knows that smoking is bad for them but here is a bit of research on the subject. Dr. H. W. Daniel, a Redding physician who specializes as an internist, reported in "The Annals of Internal Medicine" that early wrinkling is traditionally blamed on weather, aging or loss of weight but he found that none of these traditional assumptions have been proven. Daniel said he noticed the wrinkled skin of habitual cigarette smokers among his patients and set out to find whether his conclusion was correct.

In his study of 1,104 subjects, both men and women, he found that there is indeed a striking association between cigaret smoking and wrinkling of both sexes and it begins soon after age thirty. But in every age group smokers were much more prominently wrinkled than nonsmokers. Research showed that men and women smokers in the 40 to 49 age group were as wrinkled as nonsmokers of both sexes in the 60 to 69 age group.

If you think you can smoke only while you're young then quit and beat the wrinkle game forget it. Dr. Daniel said it was particularly interesting that non-smokers who had smoked while they were young showed more prominent wrinkling than total non-smokers.

There are 1400 additives used to flavor or moisten tobacco, some are dangerous when burned. The American Council on Science & Health says cocoa, licorice extract, menthol, carmel and other tobacco additives are harmless in food and beverages but produce dangerous compounds when burned.

So without a doubt, research has proven that breathing clean air is vital to delaying wrinkles because clean air brings the needed oxygen to the body's cells.

Some pessimists will say air is bad all over, so I

might as well smoke. This is the type of widespread negative thinking that corrupts our beautiful planet. If we had the proper amount of clean air and we were basically happy with ourselves then we wouldn't be so negative. So wherever we can, in whatever way we are able, we must try to improve conditions. And certainly we can't do that by adding our own personal smoke pollution.

And if all this hasn't convinced you to stop smoking or never start let me just add a few more details. Smoking uses up the Vitamin C in the body and is not only a cancer causing agent for the lungs and mouth but is also bad for the heart, eyes, nervous system, blood pressure, pulse, lower extremities and the functioning of that all important part of our bodies called the brain. Tobacco leaves are sprayed with poisonous chemicals and sometimes the spraying is done several different times adding more toxic chemicals to the nicotine, tar and lead already present. All these toxins are accumulative in the body. Also, one of the elements in tobacco that makes it so addicting is sugar; tobacco is usually sugar cured. Every skin doctor I have questioned has said emphatically that smoking deteriorates the body cells and accelerates aging in human skin.

If you want to quit smoking I'll tell you an old fashioned remedy that helped my father quit. He bought some ginger root, cut it into little quarter inch squares then put it in a dish with some water and set it in the refrigerator. Everytime he had an urge to smoke a cigarette he would take one of those little squares of ginger root and suck on it or chew it. It seemed to quench his desire for the devil weed and he quit smoking.

Then when he started gaining weight because people do tend to substitute food for cigarettes, he again used the little ginger squares but this time to curb his appetite. Ginger is a very strong root and a little goes a long way so again moderation is the key word here.

There has been a major breakthrough in utilizing Vitamin C in the human body. The key to the optimum benefits of Vitamin C is in a product called Ester C — with metabolites.

Typically, ordinary Vitamin C passes through the body with at least 78 - 88% of its nutrients potentially wasted. The ingenious folks at the Inter-Cal Corporation have clearly solved the problem of sending this crucial vitamin "down the drain."

A metabolite is a compound metabologically derived from a nutrient and usually is created in the body.

Jonathan V. Wright, M.D. of the Meridian Clinical Laboratory in Kent, Washington, has released the results of a human utilization study comparing Ester C to traditional Vitamin C. The results were mind-boggling! Ester C was consistently four times more biologically available, and after 24 hours, showed levels four times higher in the white blood cells with only one-third as much Vitamin C being excreted.

Doctors all over the world are using Ester C in nutritional therapy — and the results are outstanding.

Ester C is a registered trademark of the Inter-Cal Corporation located in Prescott, Arizona. Their scientific and medical board consists of many distinguished doctors and PhD's — Jeffrey Bland, formerly of the Linus Pauling Institute, has held International Press Conferences on the health benefits of this unique Vitamin C discovery.

Vitamin C is easily destroyed as foods are processed. Vitamin C is lost when exposed to air, heat and alkalinity. Vitamin C is depleted through long storage, soaking and slow dehydration.

Food sources of Vitamin C are: citrus fruits, strawberries, papayas, cantaloup, acerola cherries, currants, guavas, rosehips, parsley, kale, broccoli, green peppers and Brussels sprouts.

Vitamin C is a strong immunity-booster, helps reduce cholesterol, and helps prevent lesions on the walls of the blood vessels which can lead to hardening of the arteries. Drugs, over-the-counter and prescription alike including aspirin and barbiturates, lower the ascorbic acid levels in the blood. Convenience foods have much of the Vitamin C processed out and deprive the body of vitamins. Dr. Linus Pauling, the "father of Vitamin C," says that all hospital patients — no matter what illness — should be getting large does of Vitamin C every day. Vitamin C produces natural killer-cells, the first line of defense of the human body.

I personally take Ester C every day and recommend it to all my friends — yes, and I don't leave home without it!

MENTAL ATTITUDE

Dr. A.A. Chaplan, a respected psychiatrist in the Los Angeles area, had this to say about mental attitude and wrinkles:

"One's state of mind translates into body potentials whether one is aware of that or not.

"Experience with Biofeedback shows that people who often say they are relaxed are in fact tense when the actual muscle action potentials are measured. So you cannot gage your muscle relaxation from the 'Mental State' you think you experience. And, since the face is in effect a sheet of muscles interwoven to provide various functions with the skin overlying it, one must take into consideration whether these muscles are tense or not. We are dealing with interlocking mechanisms. If we are in pain we tense, if we tense too long we frown, or cause lines to appear, on the face. When we worry we furrow our brows. If we see our brows furrowed we worry, that's when the lines become indelible.

"Most people think that all sleep is a state of relaxation and release from tension, yet, in fact, many people will have seizures, heart attacks, grind their teeth and sometimes mentally fight devils thus wake up feeling as though they had wrestled alligators. This is because what is on one's mind during the day, and can be masked while the eyes are open, will come to the forefront when the eyes are closed and the subconscious is undistracted.

"Even if something is taken to induce sleep it will put the brain to sleep but not necessarily the body and one can again awaken more tired than when one went to sleep.

"Composure, serenity, inner-peace, equanimity are terms that convey the goal one seeks to combat the wear and tear of our everyday living. Certainly mental attitude has a great deal to do with this and this has a great deal to do with the wrinkles that age our faces."

The farthest distance you will ever travel in this world is the space between your ears.

CHAPTER 2

Humor & Health

Can we talk? I mean sincerely. It's not easy to be sane in an insane world but just for the health of it you have to keep laughing. For instance, it was a typical smoggy day in Los Angeles, and by the way smog destroys the body's resistance to fight disease but that's just part of the everyday aggravation. On this particular day the clock radio woke me at 6 a.m. saying, "There were 74 children hurt when a bomb exploded in a Cokeville, Wyoming school."

My first thought was "Terrorists in Wyoming?"

But no, it was just two local loonies demanding 300 million for lunch money. The bomb went off, but fortunately the only two killed were the loonies.

The next news: Moscow was admitting 13 had died from their nuclear power plant disaster but an American doctor was saying thousands could be added to that death list, still the men in charge were already talking about another plant to replace the mess. The local joke, "What's the weather in Kiev? Overcast and 10,000 degrees!"

Then I got up to read the paper and learned many bus drivers were high on drugs or alcohol and God knows what the truck drivers were doing but mechanical checks were showing more than half the trucks on the highways were unsafe.

Unsafe maintenance was also the cause of a 9 million dollar government lawsuit against Eastern Airlines and added to that came the word from air traffic controllers that the skies were out of control and not friendly anymore.

The government was saying Eastern's nuts and bolts weren't too tight. A controller was saying our radar systems were outdated and a politician was saying replacing them all at once was cost prohibitive but our President wanted to go ahead and spend billions for star wars. Who said money wasn't more valuable than lives?

Of course there were incidents of child molesting and wife beating but that was almost daily news. The final story I read was about a country and western singer, Johnny Paycheck, seems he had been found guilty of shooting a man in a bar and was sentenced to 9½ years.

Well, I thought, now instead of singing, "You can take this job and shove it," he could sing you can take this life and shove it.

But it was just another typical day of bombing, killing, child abuse, wife beating, careless workmanship and incompetence.

Please, let me hear something positive, if not positive then at least funny. I have always felt that a laugh a day keeps the doctor away and since Norman Cousins' book, "Anatomy of an Illness" was published even a lot of doctors had come to believe that humor could restore health and help to maintain it on a daily basis.

A good laugh, like a good workout, produces an overall sense of well-being says Dr. William F. Fry Jr., an associate clinical professor of psychiatry at the Stanford University Medical School.

Laughter raises skin temperature and heart rate, flexes the diaphragm, chest and abdominal muscles, exercises the shoulders, neck and face and releases adrenaline like hormones called catecholamines. These stimulate the brain, increase alertness and ready the body for action. Dr. Fry says he didn't get much agreement from other health professionals until Mr. Cousins wrote in his book that watching Marx Brothers movies and reruns of Candid Camera along with mega-doses of Vitamin C helped him recover from a degenerative spinal condition.

Many experts in the medical profession remain skeptical and want more studies done but in the meantime the rest of us who aren't experts can keep laughing because we don't need a study to know it makes us feel better.

The only doctor I know who could laugh about his profession was the medical heretic, the late Dr. Robert Mendelsohn. He kept his sense of humor, told it like it is, and advised all of us to know more than our doctors just to protect ourselves from our doctors!

Humor is healthy and even sick jokes can sometimes help. It does seem crazy to laugh at disaster but when you are totally helpless to do anything about it then humor can save your sanity when total frustration sets in. As for being obscene, tasteless and irreverent, well every comedian fits that description at one time or another or they would be carpenters instead of comedians.

I've been writing and lecturing about health for approximately 10 years and sometimes if I feel an audience drifting away when I get to a technical explanation I might insert a little shock humor. A "Pick a Finger," Joan Rivers type of humor certainly gets attention. For instance, smokers don't want to hear that they should quit smoking so I might say, "Cancer's good for you, keep smoking!"

Most people like to think that they have absolute control over their lives. That they are the ones who can smoke and not get cancer or any other myriad of diseases connected to it. When they get sick, they are sometimes so overwhelmed they can't cope, then joking is a very healthy reaction. It helps with the psycho-physiological problems that cause breakdowns in the immune system.

For instance, in 1957, a midwestern farming community discovered that the town fool, a 51 year old man had been killing local women and the ghoulish details horrified the townsfolk. Most felt the horror was too awful to joke about but thinking about it persisted and local physicians reported an outbreak of stress related problems such as hives, flu and gastrointestinal complaints. The few who told "sick jokes" were the ones who stayed healthy. Joking relieved the tension.

CHAPTER 3

Breakdowns and the Immune System

As stated in Chapter 2, humor is the ability to override really negative things, to let go of hostility or guilt and to be able to play with them. Nobody, no matter who they are, lives a life free of pain but one can cope with pain if one doesn't lose their sense of humor. Sick jokes are not the sickest reaction to horror, the sickest reaction is to have a mental and/ or physical breakdown.

Breakdowns affect the immune system and the immune system is now really in the spotlight with the widespread fear of Acquired Immune Deficiency Syndrome. In a recent lecture, I started by saying, "Sex can be hazardous to your health. In fact, given current statistics, one wonders if sex of any kind is safe. As strong a drive as sex is, it is not worth dying for."

The room always gets quiet then because nearly everyone is interested in safe sex. Whether one is heterosexual, homosexual, bisexual, non-sexual or undecided this is certainly the worst time of all for sexual guilt. Guilt causes stress and stress attracts disease and disease is rampant everywhere. Not only because of the personal pollution we might put our bodies through with bad health habits but also as discussed, because the world's atmosphere is more polluted with toxic fallout from atomic plants, chemical spraying of our food and soil and dumping hazardous materials without proper safety precautions. I wonder about the mentality of the people who do this and why they don't understand they are really contaminating their own nest.

But, getting back to the immune systems we must clearly understand that sexual guilt is very much connected to our well-being. One Sunday a friend of mine took me to a Science of Mind Church in West Hollywood. The pastor had gotten a reputation for telling it like it is. I walked in to hear her say, "Let's stop being so judgmental of each other. God loves you no matter what your personal sexual preference might be as long as you are not hurting anybody else or yourself. Today this means being very intelligent with your body and practicing safe sex. If you are a good, clean, honest, loving, person trying to do your best then you are loved by God. We are defined by the way we treat ourselves and by the way we treat other people. If you live by that golden rule then really it isn't anybody's business who's pushing your 'pee-pee' around!"

Well, that sentence brought the house down with laughter. It was like a relief valve for all the emphasis put on sex. Humor kept the pastor's congregation tuned into the sermon.

Today more people are looking for a church of "What's Happening Now." Preaching the old-fashioned 'fire and brimstone' from the pulpit never did work well in keeping people in line and it does not help us cope with today because today the promise of tomorrow is too "iffy."

It's not easy to be sane in an insane world, but in order to cope, both mind and body have to be well. Staying well is worth the effort because the effort allows you to have a healthy life in your pursuit of happiness while you are visiting this planet. It's a short visit but quality is always more desirable than quantity.

BODY AND HEADACHE

Whenever you have an ache anywhere from head to toe, it is a signal that your body chemistry is not balanced and it needs your help to right itself.

Stomach pains and acid indigestion can be as simple as not eating properly or eating too many acid foods which are meats, fish, poultry, eggs and grains. Proper balance with the alkaline forming foods; fruits, vegetables, beans and dairy are a simple solution without resorting to acid indigestion pills which often put stress on the body from the chemicals they contain.

Sometimes body aches or headaches can be caused by constipation. A clogged colon could be throwing toxins into the bloodstream. In that case, don't take an aspirin, take an enema. The proper procedure for this is in the chapter on colonics and enemas.

The Cancer Control Society often hands out leaflets called, "The American Death Ceremony." The following is what they say:

"The death ceremony started as a crude ritual, back in the days of witchcraft. In recent years it has been developed into a science. It usually takes from 10 to 15 years; however, modern scientific advancements are shortening this period of time.

"It starts with one simple aspirin for a simple headache. When one aspirin will no longer cover up the headache, take two; when two no longer cover up the headache, you take one of the stronger compounds. By this time it becomes necessary to take something for the ulcers that have been caused by the aspirin. Now that you are taking two medicines you have a good start. After a few months these medications will disrupt your liver function. If an infection develops you can take penicillin.

"Of course the penicillin will damage your red blood corpuscles and spleen so that you develop anemia. Another medication is taken to cover up the anemia. By this time all of these medications will put such a strain on your kidneys they should break down. It is now time to take some antibiotics.

"When these destroy your natural resistance to disease, you can expect a general flare-up of all your symptoms. The next step is to cover up all these symptoms with sulfa drugs. When the kidneys finally plug up, you can have them drained. Some poisons will build up in your system but you can keep going quite a while this way.

By now the medications will be so confused they won't know what they are supposed to be doing, but it doesn't really matter. If you have followed every step as directed you can now make an appointment with your undertaker.

"This game is played by practically all Americans, except for the few ignorant souls who follow nature."

By Dr. L.I.

For more information, you may send a $2.00 donation to the Cancer Control Society, 2043 No. Berendo, Los Angeles, CA 90027. Lorraine Rosenthal, co-founder, will be happy to send you a packet which contains doctor and clinic referrals for alternative therapies, a patient list, a cancer book list and dates for future cancer conventions and cancer clinic tours.

Now for arthritis there are many helpful remedies. The following is one that has helped some people I know:

1. No meat or shell fish but scale fish three times a week.

2. Use Kelp in place of salt.

3. Three colonics. One a day the first three days or take a colon cleanser with psyllium husks for five days.

4. Two tablespoons of Cod Liver Oil a day.

5. Two tablespoons raw unpasteurized Apple Cider Vinegar in a pint of hot water and sip throughout the day.

6. Six glasses of distilled water a day.

7. Take supplements, Vitamin C, 1000 mg. to 3000 mg. and one B Complex daily, plus Kyolic garlic powder capsules with calcium and Ester C, four to five a day. Plus Kyolic Liquid Garlic with B1 and

B 12 or 6 Kyolic Liquid capsules.

8. One baked red or white potato three times a week.

9. Buttermilk for a beverage but no alcohol or candy. Limit intake of caffeine.

PMS and MENOPAUSE

There seems to be a plethora of remedies recommended these days for the female miseries of PMS and menopause. Everything from vitamin, mineral, herbs and homeopathic supplements to an electric type mechanism worn around the waist that suppresses the pain of PMS. Some doctors prescribe the contraceptive pill for sufferers of PMS but this has only helped a small percentage. Also eliminating salt, sugar and caffeine from ones diet often relieves PMS symptoms.

PRE-MENSTRUAL TENSION (PMT)

It is estimated that over 30 million women presently have PMT. There are certain factors that increase the risk of having PMT — they are stress, diet, lack of physical activity, age, marital status and hormonal imbalance.

Dr. Guy E. Abrams, M.D., in his book *Pre-Menstrual Blues,* identifies four major subgroups of the typical PMT patient. They are PMT Patient A, H, C and D, as follows:

PMT Patient A — Eighty percent of these patients go through mood-swings, irritability and tension.

PMT Patient H — Over sixty percent of these PMT patients go through weight gain, swelling, bloating and tenderness of lower abdomen and breasts.

PMT Patient C — Forty percent of PMT patients of this group are characterized by craving sweets and having an increase in appetite.

PMT Patient D — Twenty percent of these patients go through pre-menstrual depression, withdrawal, confusion, crying easily, insomnia and forgetfulness.

Here are some of Dr. Abrams' suggestions for overcoming this monthly problem:

Diet — Increase intake of magnesium. Magnesium helps keep calcium in the bones where it belongs. Magnesium decreases the need for calcium, and calcium increases the need for magnesium. Dr. Abrams believes that magnesium is a mineral often deficient in American women. Dairy products have ten times more calcium than magnesium.

Limit your coffee, tea and chocolate because these substances increase the demand for B Vitamins and cause breast problems.

Limit your intake of alcohol, as it depletes the body of important nutrients and decreases the availability of sugar from the liver, leading to hypoglycemic attacks.

Increase your intake of complex carbohydrates, which are found in vegetables, legumes, beans and whole grains.

Limit the use of tobacco, fats, dairy, refined sugars, salt, chocolate and red meat.

Exercise — but not strenuous or violent exercise. The best form during this critical time of the month is walking at a fast pace in fresh air under the morning sunlight for 30 - 40 minutes. A good daily walk improves general well-being and releases tension. The popular TV program, "20-20", revealed that exercise was one of the most important ways to help reverse the aging process.

There is a product on the market called "RELEAF" for alleviating the symptoms of PMS. RELEAF is an *all-natural* product made from herbs and Vitamin B6.

Over 2,000 women who tried this formula found it to be the most effective in getting relief from the following symptoms of PMS:

cramps	depression
pain	fluid retention
headache	irritability
fatigue	physical sensitivity
lack of concentration	sleeplessness

Testing the effectiveness of RELEAF was very easy because it was taken only when symptoms occurred and was effective in 20-40 minutes. A woman didn't have to wait until she understood the cause of PMS and what she could do about it — she took this product and found relief quickly.

RELEAF works on the principle that it increases circulation to the brain and muscles, thus relieving stress and tension. Fatigue and depression dissipate when the increased blood supply is furnished to the brain and muscles, and fluid retention responds to the increased circulation of the lymphatic system (the largest organ of elimination in the body).

RELEAF is best taken when the symptons arrive with 8-10 oz. of water. Usually within 20-40 minutes the cramping, headaches, fatigue, back pain, flashes, anxiety and depression are gone. It's almost like a miracle. It is distributed by the Women's Health Institute and is made of all natural products for the betterment of women's health. RELEAF is truly Mother Nature's gift to women (and for some men too).

DUAL GARD is another excellent product from the Women's Health Institute. It is a nutritional supplement for those suffering from systemic yeast infection.

Diet does affect your moods. Judith Wurtman, Ph.D., a research scientist in the department of brain and cognitive science at the Massachusetts Institute of Technology studied the relationship of food and mood for seven years.

Dr. Wurtman concluded that carbohydrates make you sleepy, protein increases your alertness and fat dulls your ability to perform physically and mentally!

CHAPTER 4
Candida Albicans

A health problem that seems to plague more people lately is Candida Albicans. Most of the 50 or more fungi that can cause human disease are in yeast form. Candida is the most common of these because it is a normal inhabitant of all of us. It lives in our intestinal tract and is a yeast like organism. Normally, it is not a problem. However, with the use of birth control pills and various antibiotics, and/or long periods of stress; infections such as Candida, also known as moniliasis or thrush can result in both superficial disease in healthy persons and wide spread disease in patients with compromised resistance.

At its worst, Candida can cause c. endocanditis, C. Meningitis and encephalitis. But the most common symptoms are depression, fatigue, general irritation, mouth thrush and vaginitis. Clinical studies have shown that the symptoms of Candida infections can mimic anything from allergies and eye infections to colitis. The drugs commonly used against this fungus, i.e. Amphotericin B, Flucytosine and Nystatin can have adverse side effects such as kidney damage, nausea, rashes and fever.

Because of the side effects of chemical drugs, there has been a growing interest in the use of garlic as a natural fungistat. Garlic is both antifungal and antibacterial with no side effects. But, eating a lot of raw garlic could irritate the stomach. However, the proper amount and the proper kind of garlic has been shown to interfere with the reproduction and growth of fungus without affecting the host organism. Because of its non-toxicity and natural bacteriostatic properties, garlic serves as an ideal replacement for drugs used to fight fungal infections.

It is also wise to follow a yeast free diet and concentrate more on vegetables, whole grains (not wheat) low fat meat and fish. It has also been helpful to put good bacteria into the body by taking acidophilus either liquid or powder. One of the more potent ones is Kyodophilus. This helps the good bacteria fight the bad bacteria.

For the first two months, eating foods that help fight Candida is a wise idea. Vegetables should be raw, steamed or in soups. Nuts and seeds should be freshly shelled to avoid mold contamination. Avoid pistachios and peanuts. Sprouted seeds are acceptable. However, some individuals with severe Candidas must avoid nuts altogether at least for the first two months. Whole grains such as millet, rice, oats, oat bran, rice cakes, potato flour and amaranth flour are good. Some people can tolerate buckwheat, rye and barley but each person has to decide what is right for them. Generally dairy products should be eliminated for the first two months. Soy, tofu, tempeh, rice or almond milk can be substituted. Lowfat meats, poultry, fish and eggs are acceptable provided you can buy them without hormones or steroids. Shelton products are good.

Olive oil, safflower, sesame and sunflower oil are fine in limited quantities. Seaweed products, miso and taheebo tea are good. Soaking fruits and vegetables in a dilute solution of water and plain household bleach — 1 tsp. bleach in a ½ gallon of water to kill yeast and pesticides is good. Some people prefer to use salt and lemon juice or salt and vinegar to clean fruits and veggies.

CANDIDA

The following is a personal experience of one womans problem with Candida. Her name is Vickie.

"It is my belief my problems with Candida began many years ago; however, in 1984 I started to experience severe menstrual pain and suffered from numerous bladder infections, which became progressively worse. For 10 years I had taken birth control pills and experienced a vaginal discharge for the past 4 years. Over the last 1½ years I had been treated with tetracycline in very high doses along with other hormones to correct my hormone imbalances.

A laparoscopy revealed a benign tumor and endometriosis, resulting in a total hysterectomy and extensive bladder repair. Two weeks later I was again hospitalized for widespread infection. During this time I was given five different antibiotics, some of them repeatedly. Soon after, a series of strange symptoms listed below manifested themselves.

Pounding in my head, headaches, strange visual disturbances, numbness and a tingling sensation, fluid in my eyes, extreme fatigue, confusion, clicking noises, spots in front of my eyes, dizziness, no coordination, severe sinus problems, poor memory, a slight chronic yeast infection.

My gynecologist kept increasing my estrogen dosage in an attempt to alleviate some of the symptoms but to no avail. Life was becoming increasingly difficult. When the pounding in my head could be heard over the noise in a room full of people, a neurologist was consulted. His concern was the possibility of an artery malfunction and insisted on performing a brain cat scan. This procedure called for dye to be injected into my veins. During the cat scan my throat swelled shut and my heart beat became irregular. Adrenalin and other medications were given to try and counteract the allergic reaction to the dye. From that day forward, allergic reactions started to develop with almost every chemical I came in contact with. Gradually many different foods would also bring on typical asthmatic symptoms.

No arterial problems showed up in the cat scan so an ear specialist was recommended. He could not find any reason for the pulsating and other symptoms but felt a possible aneurysm might be the problem and wanted to do an angiogram. I refused after my experience with the brain cat scan.

I just happened upon Dr. John Trowbridge's

book on Candida, entitled "The Yeast Syndrome," published by Bantam Books, and for the first time read of other people with symptoms similar to mine. I put myself on his recommended diet and made an appointment to see an allergist/clinical ecologist working with Candida patients. In the meantime, I was still seeking an answer to the pounding in my head. The ear specialist suggested seeing an orthodontic TMJ specialist because I had been told years before I had a misalignment of the jaw. The TMJ problem was verified and they started me on a corrective orthodontic program to pull my jaw back into its proper position. However, after two adjustments using liquid acrylic on the mouthpiece, I had such severe allergic reactions we had to abandon the corrective treatment.

As a patient of the allergy specialist I submitted a blood specimen to a California lab which revealed I had a Candida count of 41.7. Normal is approximately 10. The doctor felt this was a considerable amount of Candida. I continued on Trowbridge's program even to the extent of cuting out fruits and grains. Vitamin, minerals, evening primrose oil, linseed oil, Nystatin, garlic oil perles and yeast vaccine shots were started. I contacted the author of a Candida cookbook and asked what she would suggest to keep me from losing additional weight. She suggested adding more oils and butter to my diet. I increased my garlic oil capsules from eight to twelve per day.

Each passing week, my food and allergy sensitivities were getting worse. I had to take a leave of absence from work due to the installation of new carpet (using glue) in the building. My sensitivities now included: inks and carbons, fertilizers, household cleaners, synthetic fabrics, candles, waxes, chlorine, pollen, mold and mildew, insecticides, laundry detergents, cosmetics, food coloring, burning wood, grass, all tobacco, plastics and vinyls, weed killers, soaps, perfume, colognes, paint, varnish, coal, trees.

Trying to keep all of these substances out of my environment was impossible, even though I had nearly stripped my home.

By the middle of June, my weight was down to 79 pounds and I was really desperate. The Nystatin relieved to a small degree the numbness, tingling and headaches but everything else kept getting worse. Beef and broccoli were the only food I could still tolerate and I was eating them three times a day. My fatigue was extreme and I spent most days confused, crying and looking for an answer to this illness.

It was then I saw an ad in a health magazine for a liquid garlic and wondered if it might be more effective than the garlic oil capsules. I called the company and received the address and telephone number of a clinic that successfully treats not only Candida, but illness of all kinds, using a natural diet which included liquid Kyolic garlic. After two weeks at this clinic, I felt like a new person. I threw away all medications, estrogen, etc. My mental confusion was 90% better, and I gained 8 pounds. My food and chemical sensitivities improved little by little. I returned to work in one month and was totally free of any allergies in two months. I continued to feel better each day and now have more energy than I ever remember. After four months, another yeast count was taken and it had dropped to the normal range. My doctor was very surprised, to say the least, that anyone could reduce their yeast count so quickly.

The health recovery program I was taught consisted of an unusual vegetarian diet, and stressed the importance of exercise, rest, fresh air, sunlight and pure water. Among other things, I learned at the bottom of every illness is an improperly functioning digestive system. Restoring your digestive system through the basic principles of this program will restore good health. This program has been used extensively in reconditioning centers in this country and around the world to restore health and for the prevention of disease.

As we can see diet is just as important as any supplements we might take. Basically when one has Candida, it is best to have no meats, oils, sugar or dairy until the body is well and back in balance again.

Vickie has become her own nutritional researcher but in order to get well she went to Nancy Burnett, a Nutritional Researcher at 114 W. Main St., Cottonwood, Arizona, (602) 634-2017. Tapes are available.

Nancy Burnett is the innovator of the "New-Start Diet" that has literally saved hundreds of lives. Nancy's program consists of 16 one-hour tapes. Her program is drug-free . . . no nystalin and no yeast vaccines . . . not too many supplements, but is based on a well-conceived program of diet and exercise. These tapes may be ordered from Nancy Burnett.

Nancy is an ex-policewoman who was active in drug enforcement in Arizona and gave up her career to dedicate her life to helping the unfortunate victims of Candida albicans. Her program has also saved the lives of many drug addicts, manic depressives, alcoholics, etc. Nancy's theory is, "change your diet, change your life." Nancy is a dynamic, healthy lady who inspires one to achieve a higher sense of well-being. She has given of her time unselfishly, and is loved by all who have come in contact with her.

YEAST GUARD

A major breakthrough in vaginal yeast infection is the introduction to the United States of Yeast-Gard. Yeast-Gard was formulated in Canada and used successfully in clinical trials with over 3,000 women.

Yeast'Gard brings quick relief from itching, burning and irritation, eliminates unpleasant discharge and most important of all kills vaginal yeast infections.

Yeast-Gard is a natural product, it has no side effects, it does not require a doctor's prescription. It is convenient to use and inexpensive to buy. It comes with a special applicator and 10 suppositories.

Traditional treatments for yeast vaginities simply don't work for many women, especially those who have suffered for years.

"Yeast-Gard is a product that offers hope for millions of women who now suffer needlessly. When it is incorporated in a treatment program that addresses the true cause of their problems, women can look to a lifetime of comfort and better health."

Yeast-Gard is now called Femicine in California.

John Parks Trowbridge, M.D.
Co-author of the best selling book
THE YEAST SYNDROME
published by Bantam Books

DUAL GUARD

DUAL-GARD presents the best of herbal medicine and garlic research. DUAL-GARD is especially formulated for those suffering intestinal yeast infections.

It is the perfect nutritional supplement to take for those suffering from systemic yeast infections.

It slowly builds the body's own natural defenses to overcome the yeast syndrome.

DUAL-GARD is a special combination of Kyolic Odorless Garlic Extract with superior food enzymes; Ester-C, a more potent form of Vitamin C; Eichinecca, Beta Carotene, Taheboo Bark, Astragulus Root, Black Walnut, Cascara Sagrada Bark and Kyo-Dophidus, a superior lactic bacteria product. DUAL-GARD, in combination with a diet free of oils, sugar, dairy, meat and fowl and a diet high in complex carbohydrates (beans, grains), plus green vegetables, has done more for bringing Candida albicans to its knees than all the drugs and vaccines can ever do. Only the body heals, and nutritional support is what gives the body the energy to do what it does best — defend itself.

Candida albican is a troublesome medical problem that affects 30% of the population. The A,B,C, and D of Candidasis are caused by: (A) over-use of antibiotics, (B) birth control pills, (C) cortisone and (D) a deplorable diet.

Four excellent books on the subject include, "THE YEAST SYNDROME" by Dr. John Parks Trowbridge, and Dr. Morton Walker published by Bantam Books.

"Candida" by Dr. Luc DeShepper.

"The Yeast Connection" by Dr. William Crook.

"Candida-Free, You and Me" by JoAnn Rohn.

The first three books are available at most health food stores and bookstores, and the book by JoAnn Rohn can be ordered directly from the Holistic Living Center, 109 West Beaver, Fort Morgan, Colorado 80701, phone (303) 867-4852.

CHAPTER 5

Hospitals

When aches and pains get bad enough that you have to go to a hospital you should be aware of your patient rights. I discussed this with D. Rivellino Walsh, a hospital administrator for 20 years at Misericardia Medical Center, New York and Los Robles Medical Center, Thousand Oaks, Calif. and she agreed that patients need to participate more in their own health care. Ms. Walsh was also an administrator at the Jules Stein Institute in Los Angeles for seven years. The following is her patient awareness list:

1. Patients have the right to all their records at any time.

2. Patients have the right to refuse any test they feel is not right for them, unless they are thoroughly explained and this includes the drawing of blood.

3. Your armband must be checked before a medication, test or procedure is given.

4. The anesthesist should be seen or talked with 24 hours prior to elective surgery. Naturally this is not possible with emergency surgery. A patient has the right to discuss the type of anesthetic to be used after the options and dangers of each type are outlined.

5. You have the right to know what medications you are taking and what, if any, adverse reactions or side effects there might be. The standard reply of "Just something the doctor ordered!" is not good enough.

6. Every patient has the right to discuss food needs with a dietician and/or nutritionist, especially if on a restricted diet.

7. Patients must demand from a physician a full explanation of their diagnosis and prognosis and what kind of alternative treatments are available.

8. A patient has the right to ask for a second opinion. A referral should not come from the primary physician.

9. Specialists and general practitioners should be board certified plus they should be certified yearly with continuing education programs. To find out if a doctor is board certified look on their wall for a Board Certified degree, if you don't see it then ask and if you are in doubt then call the Board of Medical Examiners.

10. Radiology (X-Rays) should be kept to a minimum. This includes mammography. Unless a woman is in a high risk group I would not

recommend an annual mammography just because she is over 40. However, self-examination and/or physician examination is recommended. And, by expressing concern to your physician you may find that alternative tests are possible. Most tests are performed for the convenience of the physician and hospital staff.

11. When having implants you have the right to know what risks are involved, i.e. mechanical failures or other potential problems. You can also ask for a list of former patients that have the implant and if it is possible to talk with some of them.

12. Prior to admission be aware of a hospitals reputation. When was the last accreditation given. Any known problems? All technicians should be trained and registered, i.e. R.N., L.P.N. You might want to go in ahead of time, introduce yourself and find out who will be caring for you. Don't just assume that if someone is on staff they have been checked.

13. At the time of discharge ask for a completely itemized bill. The most common problem is when patients are charged for items that were never used. Even if you have insurance, do not feel that the insurance company is paying for it because ultimately YOU PAY for it in higher insurance rates.

Ms. Walsh further explained that on an average a prep tray cost $40. Sheepskins are $50 and can be taken home with you. Sheepskins are put under a patient who has surgery so the patient doesn't get bedsores.Cloth leg splints are about $60 and are also reusable. The basic hospital cost only pays for your room and board (meals). Each test should be signed by the patient. This helps the patient become fully aware of what each test is taken for.

Your health is YOUR RESPONSIBILITY. It is unwise to check yourself into a hospital like you might drop your car off at a repair shop.

Four out of 10 hospitalizations during a recent 7-year period were avoidable, according to a nationwide study by the Rand Corp.

The recently released study found that 23 percent of admissions — and about 33 percent of all days spent in the hospital — were for patients whose illnesses did not require hospitalization.

In addition, another 17 percent of hospital admissions could have been avoided by sending patients to facilities where simple surgical procedures such as dilation and curettage, bladder exams and hernia-related treatments are routinely done on an outpatient basis. The study was conducted from November 1974 through January 1982.

What causes many of the bodyaches and headaches we might have are deplorable diets and drugs (prescription and non-prescription). So when you do take a prescription or check into a hospital, make sure that the cure is not worse than the disease.

On one episode of the TV show "60 Minutes" it was revealed that hospitals expect interns to work 36 hour shifts. This expectation is ridiculous. Nobody should be expected to be mentally and physically alert for more than 8 hours. Even though they were told to take cat-naps between shifts, the body stress would still be too exhausting. So the best advice anyone could get is to always make sure any procedure or operation is absolutely necessary because putting chemicals into, or cutting into the body for any reason causes the body stress.

Dr. Robert Mendelsohn often stated that many more hysterectomies have been performed than were necessary and recently it has been reported that many more Caesarean sections are being performed than are absolutely necessary. The American College of Obstetricians and Gynecologists and a federal agency showed the Caesarean rate between 1979 and 1984 increased from 14.1% to 19% even though a U.S. government task force called for major reforms in this area more than eight years ago.

Doctors contend it is a fear of malpractice suits but critics say it is linked more to greed and convenience on the part of some physicians. The time of birth can be regulated to the physicians convenience and it also costs more to have a Caesarean. The average cost of a vaginal delivery is $1600, for a Caesarean it is approximately $2,000.

Insurance companies are now the ones requesting mandatory second opinions in some parts of the country. The medical profession knows that vaginal birth should be preferred if it can be safely accomplished because it carries none of the risks of the surgical delivery. Surgical delivery is an operation that loses two to three times the amount of blood that vaginal delivery does. Unless it is absolutely necessary, Caesarean delivery is a dangerous procedure for both mother and baby.

A competent and professional hospital staff will welcome and respect any questions you might have and the help you can offer towards your recovery.

You have a right to know what is planned or contemplated for you. A complete history of you and your allergies must be taken by the anesthesiologist prior to any surgery. A small amount of any drug to be used should be tested before the full amount is given. THIS COULD BE A LIFE SAVING PROCEDURE. A horrifying example of what could happen when this isn't done happened to the lovely and talented actress Anne Jeffreys. Anne almost lost her life because she was given a drug called Streptokinaise to clear a painful blood clot in her leg. She was not tested beforehand to see if she might be allergic to the drug and within minutes after it was administered she began the most terrifying night of her life. Anne is a dear and sweet friend and as we had lunch one afternoon about three months after it happened she told me the story.

Anne said, "The doctor told me the drug was safe and that he'd give it to his own wife but," she shook her head, "I wonder how much he loves his wife! I found out later that there is a test that can be done but this vascular surgeon told me there was no allergy test available for this drug. So I accepted what he told me and he administered the drug, then left. I was chatting and joking with the nurse when all of a sudden I felt these horrible pains, as if I was in labor. Then I started getting electrical shocks all over my body. At the same time, big red welts started popping out on my face and body as if I had been stung by a thousand bees. My face blew up like a balloon and blood started squirting like fountains, blood from my eyes, my nose, and lesions opened on the back of my neck.

I was literally bleeding to death. I told myself to

remain calm to try and keep my blood pressure down. I had to have a complete blood transfusion, using plasma and frozen blood. I'll tell you when that frozen blood hit my veins I was shivering in places I didn't know I possessed.

At one point, I felt myself slipping away. I was being sucked down this tunnel with a bright white glowing light at the end. Fortunately, my personal physician had been called in and he was sitting at my head when I weakly murmured, 'I'm leaving.' He snapped orders and helped to bring me back. If he hadn't been there I'm sure nobody would have heard me because of all the noise and confusion in the hospital. That is a pet peeve of mine about hospitals, they tell everybody to be quiet but the doctors, nurses and attendants are very careless about the chatter and noise they make. And intensive care was the worst! They put you in there because you're on the critical list and then they don't let you rest because they're always looking in on you. In the hospital I was in near Palm Springs there were no curtains on the windows in Intensive Care and the light was disturbing to my rest.

But when I felt I was going down that tunnel and leaving this life I heard a voice say, "You're not ready yet!' I was so exhausted all I wanted to do was sleep but the nurses kept waking me up to give me sleeping pills! When I refused them, well," she laughed, "they get all flustered and confused because you're going against doctors' orders. But I felt I knew what my body needed and at that point it certainly wasn't sleeping pills! When I finally got out of there, two weeks later, I felt that a hospital was not a very good place for a sick person."

Anne Jeffreys is such a loving, kind and caring person that we, her friends, her family and her fans are lucky she came back. However this is an example of what can happen if the proper precautions are not taken when chemicals are administered to the body. The side effects could be life threatening.

Let me repeat, I believe in combining medical science with homeopathic remedies. Therefore, whenever I have to have X-Rays I always increase my Vitamin C intake to 4000 mg. spaced throughout the day before and after the X-Ray. I also eat more complex carbohydrates to increase my (SOD) Superoxide Dismustase.

Don't take your health care for granted. Not all physicians are competent, just as not all car mechanics are competent. Physicians are human, capable of mistakes, however, in their position a mistake could be a life and death matter. Your most important patient right is the right to know everything that is happening to you during your health care and during hospitalization. Do not let the atmosphere or the professional staff intimidate you. Remember, a really competent and professional staff will welcome and respect any questions you might have and the help that you can offer towards your recovery.

Staying well and away from too many doctors and hospitals is part of the plan for delaying wrinkles. Recently, Dr. Richard Wenzel of the University of Virginia, reported that his findings showed hospital infections cause 4 times more deaths than traffic accidents yearly. Of approximately 38 million people who check into hospitals in America annually 2.5 million will develop infections there and 200,000 will die from them. The annual death toll from traffic accidents is roughly 50,000.

The primary responsibility of any medical person is in the medical oath; that if you can do no good then at the very least do no harm; yet conventional drugs and allopathy is based in the treatment of symptoms and uses many toxic drugs with harmful side effects, some even known to be capable of triggering cancer.

CHAPTER 6
Bodyaches

Some well known bodyaches and pains are caused by Arthritis, Rheumatism, Gout and that age old misery backache. Just about everybody gets a backache once in a while, but with most of us it goes away with time and rest. Often what causes backache is excessive exercise and/or stress and strain on back muscles.

An old fashioned grandma's remedy for backache which is still useful today is horse linament. You can usually find this at animal feed stores or veterinary offices. I think I recall one called Bigle Oil. There are also ointments like Tiger Balm and Sunbreeze Balm from Chinese remedies.

What causes Arthritis, Rheumatism and Gout? Researchers recently developed a theory that arthritis is caused by a virus-like organism. I once had gout in my left foot and I know it was caused directly from my diet which at that time was too high in Uric Acid forming foods. Or as physicians often say, foods that have very large amounts of purine bodies. Specifically, those foods are: red meats or meat extracts; sweets, liver, sweetbreads, brains, kidney; also Anchovies, Sardines in oil and meat gravies. Diet is an important factor in all body and head aches. However, there is no one diet that is good for all because everybody is different. One can only try what is recommended by the "experts" and then feel what is best for them.

There are a wide variety of drugs prescribed for Arthritis and at the top of the list is Aspirin. Aspirin reduces the inflammation associated with certain forms of arthritis, especially Rheumatoid Arthritis. Actually Aspirin was invented for treating this particular disease as it reduces swelling, stiffness and pain and is a mild sedative. A doctor should determine how much you need. However, like any drug, Aspirin has side effects that range from just irritating to life threatening. The side effects could be ringing in the ears, dizziness, headache, dimness of vision, mental confusion, nausea, vomiting and diarrhea to gastric irritation so severe that it causes internal bleeding. I have personal knowledge of this when my father almost died from internal bleeding after taking Aspirin for his Arthritis pain.

In 1983, a new type of Aspirin became available which is timed release. It is a prescription drug. Overall, Aspirin is usually safe and reliable but each individual has to find this out for themselves.

Doctors have told me that no two osteoarthritic patients have exactly the same condition and that is why there is no single drug or combination of drugs that can be used for all patients. Again Aspirin is the most widely used but two others are Phenylbutazone and Indomethacin. If your doctor recommends these ask him about side effects or get a book on drugs and look up the side effects yourself.

The most common drug used for Rheumatoid Arthritis is again Aspirin and the same drugs used for Osteoarthritis plus Cortisone, gold treatment and antimalaria drugs. As with all drugs they should be carefully monitored and regulated and patients need complete blood counts and urinalysis during the course of any treatment.

The most common drug used in the treatment of Gout is Colchicine and is produced from the Autumn Crocus. Also used are Phenylbutazone, Probenecid, Sulfinpyrazone and Allopurinol.

One of the drugs put on the market in 1982 and hailed with a lot of fanfare was a non-steroidal, anti-inflammatory one-a-day pill, Oraflex. It was pulled off the market only a few months later because of adverse side effects. Which makes one wonder . . . who do they test these pills on before they become available to the general public and why didn't they find out about the adverse side effects before issuing it? Another one-a-day pill being used now is Piroxi-cam and so far the public is being assured that it is safe.

For my own touch of gout I have used Certo liquid fruit pectin, 2 tablespoons A.M. & P.M. My friend and fellow nutritionist, Sally Kelly, told me about this simple home remedy.

HERBS

Herbs that may help in arthritic conditions include: raw garlic, kyolic odorless garlic, devil's claw, yucca, cayenne, chapparal alfalfa and celerey seed.

When pain and crippling is really severe, doctors may prescribe surgery. As with all surgery, this should be examined and analyzed before doing. Sometimes, physical therapy, exercise, proper nutrition, a positive attitude, a good sense of humor, rest and hot or cold treatments can be used effectively.

The proper balance between rest and exercise is MODERATION. Walking, not running or jogging, is still one of the best exercises known to humanity. There are arm, hand, finger, leg and feet exercises that mainly stretch the body to help circulation.

A warm, almost hot bath can be effective but is not recommended for longer than 20 minutes at a time because it could make one weak. A cold compress such as an ice bag will produce a numbing effect and give temporary relief from pain.

CHAPTER 7
Wrinkles

The next friend or enemy on the wrinkle list is the food we eat. Fortunately, as we draw to the close of the 20th century, many of us have become aware of our nutrition.

Food processors say putting preservatives in our food maintains longer shelf life. That's fine for the shelf life but does nothing to preserve our life. The best foods to eat are natural, non-processed, non-colored, without preservatives and artificial flavors.

Over the last few years many people have turned to Vegetarianism to get away from the hormones, antibiotics and preservatives injected into meats. That's a good idea if you know how to maintain body homeostasis with the proper amount of acid/alkaline balance to stay healthy. Balancing body chemistry means getting the proper amount of amino acids, vitamins and minerals to maintain our youthful appearance.

A proper balance can be accomplished with 80 percent alkaline forming foods and 20 percent acid forming foods. This would supply the necessary amounts of protein, carbohydrates, fats, liquids, vitamins and minerals.

Basically meat, fish, poultry, eggs and grains are acid forming. Fruits, vegetables, beans and dairy products are alkaline forming.

Protein builds muscle, flesh, and repairs body wear and tear. Carbohydrates (starch and sugar) supply energy and heat. Fats supply reserve energy and heat. Liquids are necessary for proper elimination. Minerals help with rebuilding and functioning of the body and are essential for well-balanced nutrition. And vitamins are the nutritive materials necessary for basic good health.

It is easily possible to be a "Junk Food Vegetarian" and even if we consciously avoid junk food our soil is now contaminated with air and water pollution and depleted from chemical sprays and pesticides. So now even our fruits and vegetables are somewhat contaminated by man's "progress." But don't get discouraged — fight back. It is possible to wash off some of these chemicals with a solution of salt and lemon juice, a teaspoon of salt and juice from half a lemon, or a solution of one tablespoon Clorox to one gallon of water and then use a scrub brush or a scrub net and rinse in clear water. It is not possible to wash off added hormones and preservatives from meats.

But digging a little deeper into our soil we find that many important nutrients are depleted from the ground because farmers don't have the time or take the time to rotate crops, give their land a rest period after a certain number of years and use natural insect repellants instead of chemicals. Farmers claim over-population has forced them to increase production and they can't afford the time it takes to do things the way Mother Nature intended them to be done. So we have soil depleted of vital nutrients and we do not get the proper amounts of vitamins and minerals from food grown in that soil. (It does seem to me that if Mother Nature planned on feeding us this way she must have assumed we would have the good sense to limit our number, something that makes Planned Parenthood seem advisable.)

The proper balance of nutrients are essential to a wrinkle free face because that helps the body avoid internal stress by keeping chemical toxins to a minimum. We fight back by taking supplements in the form of vitamins, minerals, herbs and sometimes cell salts. Or we buy wheat germ, yeast and lecithin separately to replace what should have been in our food in the first place. And of course try to buy certified organically grown foods.

SALT-FREE, UNCOOKED SAUERKRAUT

The great Russian scientist, Professor Elie Metchnikoff, was a fervent believer that good health begins in the colon. Metchnikoff believed that putrefactive bacteria are held in check by friendly lactic acid micro-organisms, called lactobacillus acidophilus, which produce lactic acid ferments detrimental to the unfriendly bacteria.

Metchnikoff's research was based upon studying the dietary habits of people from Eastern Europe living active, robust, healthy lives up to 100 years of age.

He felt that one of the most contributing factors to their longevity was the eating of foods rich in lactic acid.

Metchnikoff found one of the best sources of lactic acid in the diet of these people was their homemade, salt-free sauerkraut. It was this staple of their diet, he stated, that produced the greatest amount of friendly bacteria in the intestines.

Sauerkraut is not only rich in lactic acid but is also high in Vitamin C and enzymes plus Vitamins B1 and B2.

Because it kept so well, sauerkraut was probably one of the first health foods to travel all around the world.

Sauerkraut is a weight-watcher's delight. One cup of sauerkraut contains only 33 calories and at the same time provides the intestines with the necessary bulk, moisture and lubrication to assist one to have regular elimination.

The Germans fell in love with this perfect food, thus the Teutonic moniker for sauerkraut ("sour cabbage").

Sauerkraut adds zest and goodness to meals in an endless variety of tantalizing dishes. The perfect sauerkraut on the market today is by Vegi-Delite, and is produced by the Deer Garden Rejuvenative Foods Company, P.O. Box 8464, Santa Cruz, California 95061, phone (408) 462-6715.

Evan Richards is the creator of this super-healthful sauerkraut, using organic cabbage and raw cultured vegetables. Mr. Richards has written a book, *The Complete Guide to Raw Cultured Vegetables,* that everyone should read. In the book he explains the whole philosophy of raw cultured vegetables that can help keep the body disease-free; how raw vegetables help alleviate the negative reactions of Candida; how to make your own raw cultured vegetables; how enzymes and flora in raw vegetables make them some of the most helpful foods you can eat, and the macrobiotics of raw cultured vegetables.

While studying to obtain my Master of Science degree in Nutrition I learned that the body metabolizes natural vitamins more efficiently than synthetic ones. Research indicates that natural vitamins are superior to synthetics, even when chemical analysis shows them to be the same. It seems that our bodies know the difference even if the analysts do not. In spite of this research the FDA claims there is no difference between natural and synthetic vitamins. But to prove my point I refer to chromatography.

Chromatography is an analysis method used to literally photograph molecules of both organic and inorganic substances. Chromatographs show a distinct difference between synthetic and natural Vitamin C. Synthetic Ascorbic Acid and natural Vitamin C are chemically identical except the chromatographs of the natural Vitamin C show "impurities" which have been determined to be enzymes. Enzymes are protein factors which apparently assist in the absorption and utilization of the vitamin on a cellular level. Some vitamins are the same biochemically whether synthetic or natural but this is not true of Vitamins C and E.

Dr. Samuel Ayers, Jr. M.D. researched this and wrote an article in the August 27, 1973 issue of the "Journal of the AMA." Briefly he stated the natural Vitamin E (tocopherol) in which the alpha fraction contains virtually all the therapeutically active principles; d-Alpha-Tocopheryl Acetate is derived from natural sources; i.e. wheat germ oil, whereas dl-Alpha-Tocopherylacetate is the synthetic form. While they may appear identical the natural form is considerably more active than the (dl) form. The Animal Research Council subcommittee for Vitamin E standards has shown that the relative potency of d-alpha tocopheryl acetate is 20 percent greater than the (dl) form. Dr. Ayers said, "In order to obtain the maximum therapeutic effect from Vitamin E the physician should specify the d-alpha-tocopheryl acetate."

And on the subject of Vitamin C, I refer to British researcher, Isabel Jennings of the University College at Cambridge. She compares synthetic and natural vitamins in her book, "Vitamins in Endocrine Metabolism." She states, "The close relations, although useful in many ways, pose some problems in that they may have only a fraction, whether large or small, of the biological activity of the natural product. While synthetic Vitamin C is chemically identical to the natural vitamin and an equal effective anti-oxidant, it does not have the same value in promoting health of the capillaries."

The reason I bring up this research is that I often hear people say, "I take vitamins but they don't make any difference in the way I feel." Perhaps they're taking the wrong kind of vitamins and the body might not be metabolizing them efficiently. I feel strongly that if a person is not getting the right kind of vitamins then the health of the capillaries is affected and the body will degenerate more rapidly. Of course, degeneration of the body causes lines in the face.

As Americans we tend to think of ourselves as the healthiest people in the world but in reality the Cancer Research Institute has reported we are about 89th in world health. Our critical health care bill is approximately 400 billion dollars a year. We are 26th in longevity in the world and we have an epidemic amount of degenerative diseases like diabetes, cancer, heart disease and dental caries. It isn't so amazing that so many people have cancer today, what is amazing is that we all don't have cancer today. Our country is the most modern and progressive in the world, but as I said previously, our progress is killing us.

However, the theme of this book is to know how to fight back. Not to give in to degenerating diseases and wrinkles just because they appear to be the norm today. So I am going to give you a list of supplements and other aids that are known to help us hang in there, handle pollution and stress and delay those telltale signs of aging as long as humanly possible.

Vitamins B1, 2, 6, 12, Pantothenic Acid, Niacinamide,Vitamins E and C, Folic Acid, Choline, Inositol, Paba, Brewers Yeast which contains all the above B vitamins and added minerals. Pantothenic Acid and Vitamin B 5 have been touted by some nutritionists as a help in avoiding gray hair, dry skin and eczema. Animals given a diet deficient in Panto-thenic Acid developed those problems. The B Vita-mins are all synergistic, which means they need each other to function efficiently. Some foods rich in B vitamins are liver, yeast, egg yolk, peanuts, wheat germ and whole grains. But remember, Pantothenic Acid dissolves in water and is destroyed when Baking Soda is added to food.

Millet is rich in vitamins and minerals and has all the nutrients needed for a balanced diet. Sesame seeds and sesame oil are rich in calcium, protein and unsaturated fatty acids.

The basic food minerals are Calcium Chro-mium, Cobalt, Copper, Iron, Iodine, Magnesium, Manganese, Molybdenum, Phosphorous, Potas-sium, Selenium, Sulfur, Sodium, Zinc, Chlorine, Fluorine and Vanadium. Too much or too little of any of these could cause problems in body home-ostasis. If you suspect you might have a problem in this area then check with your doctor. There are blood tests that can be helpful.

Herbs and Cell Salts are also in the area of supplements. An entire book could be written on each subject but I will try to give a general idea on how they can be used for beneficial results and as an aid to keeping worry lines off our faces.

Certain herbs such as Kelp, Sarsparilla Root and Raw Palmetto Berries have been known to be helpful for the hot-flashes caused by menopause and for male impotence. Arthritis and rheumatism have been helped by Alfalfa, Celery Seed, Burdock Root, Garlic, Chapparal and Cayenne. Herbs reputed to help maintain weight control are Chickweed, Fennel

Seed, Burdock Root, Kelp, Bladderwrack and Chia Seeds. Herbs which have a reputation for internal cleansing are Ginger Root, Licorice Root, Butternut Bark, Rhubarb Root, Cascara Sagrada Bark, Irish Moss, Senna Leaves and Buckthorn.

When you get that "up-tight" feeling don't grab a chemical drug that could be harmful and have side effects that stress the body, take some Valerian Root. The Valerian herb is a natural tranquilizer.

The average diet is usually lacking in most of these herbs and therefore the body is not only missing their special benefits but also their nutrient value.

MINERALS

Everybody seems to know about vitamins these days but ironically very few know that without the proper amount of minerals in the body, vitamins would be useless. That's right, a body cannot function without the proper minerals no matter how many vitamins it has. Each cell of the human body contains 60 minerals, 7 are major minerals and 53 are what we call trace minerals. Minerals are essential to the body as they act as catalysts for the enzyme actions needed for every vital body function.

In the past, scientists never thought much about minerals because a very small amount was needed for the body to function in good health. Our soil was rich in all the elements we needed. Now, however, our soils are depleted from pollution, chemical sprays, non-organic fertilizers and simple over use.

Trace elements are also called micro-nutrients, the prefix "micro" meaning very small. They are distinguished from those mineral elements that are known to be required for life in large quantities and which are called macro-nutrients. The macro-nutrients are calcium, phosphorus, potassium, iron and magnesium. The imbalance of any one of these elements means trouble. The lack of any one makes life impossible. Now scientists believe that this is also true of the micronutrients such as iron, iodine, copper, manganese, zinc, cobalt, molydenum, selenium, chromium, tin and vanadium. There is also a newly discovered one called Germanium.

The Japanese have done research on Germanium and are convinced it is absolutely necessary for the human immune system. They believe it can help the body to overcome cancer, heart disease and even AIDS. Germanium stimulates the body's production of interferon which is a natural disease fighter.

One of the reasons I tout garlic so much is because it and Ginseng are the two herbs that have a high amount of Germanium in them provided they are grown in rich organic soil. Just as difficult as it is today to find good soil that is how difficult it is to find good clean oxygen. Germanium carries extra oxygen into the body. Germanium carries oxygen to places in your body where oxygen from your lungs is in short supply. Tests have shown that cancer grows only in the absence of oxygen. It is interesting to note that almost every chemical drug available on the market today decreases the amount of oxygen in the body. In America it is illegal to cure anything with a substance other than an approved drug. However, in Japan Germanium is known to be successful in the treatment of a broad range of problems including arthritis, osteoporosis, hepatitis, cancer, leukemia, cataracts, liver disease and heart disease. It is said to retard aging by balancing free-radical metabolism.*

Farm practices which influence the quality of the soil and the crop should be the concern of every human being who isn't growing his own food. We need to eat organically grown food in order to remain healthy throughout life but in the last half of the 20th Century it has become exceedingly difficult to do so and that is why most of us have to supplement our diets with vitamins, minerals, herbs, cell salts, flower remedies and any other natural help we can get. One product that contains all the macro and micro minerals in liquid form is called Body Toddy, it is processed and distributed by The Rockland Corp. 12215 E. Skelly Dr. Tulsa, OK 74128. The minerals come from a large prehistoric plant deposit and therefore are basically formulated by "Mother Nature" who seems to know better than anybody what's good for us.

*The Report on Germanium by Karl Loren
Life Extension Educational Service
1759 Cosmic Way
Glendale, CA 91201

IRON

The white blood cells of the immune system use iron, along with Vitamin C to zap invading germs. Iron absorption is enhanced by Vitamin C and both supplements should be taken at the same time. One out of every three people in the population consume 25% less iron than they should. For women the figure is even higher — 33%. Even a 10% dietary shortage can depress the immune system.

Iron in the blood is what enables us to breathe. It is part of the hemoglobin, the substance which continously carries oxygen from the lungs to all parts of the body and brings back unwanted carbon dioxide to the lungs to exhale. Iron promotes this process. If there is no iron — there is no hemoglobin. Iron is present in every living cell and is the most important of all the trace minerals to obtain in adequate amounts in the food we eat. Iron is one of the most poorly absorbed minerals. It is impossible for pregnant women and women of childbearing age to obtain adequate amounts of iron from the average diet. Iron deficiency can pose serious health problems for athletes as iron is lost through sweating.

Fortunately there is a product on the market called "IRON POWER*," an herbal invigorating iron tonic in liquid or tablet form. IRON POWER comes highly recommended because it is non-constipating and an effective way to increase your iron intake. It is also fortified with Vitamin C and the B complex.

You can depend on IRON POWER for substantial absorption of organic iron in the blood and utilization for oxygen transport and other vital purposes. Getting adequate amounts of iron is most important during the growing years, during pregnancy, while nursing, during periods of convalescence and during times of imbalanced diets. IRON POWER helps fight fatigue naturally.

IRON POWER is made by Salus-Haus of Germany, a world leader in natural sources of herbs and food supplements. IRON POWER is available at health food stores in the United States and Canada and the liquid IRON POWER tastes great.

*Iron Power is the same formula as Floradix.

Dandelion greens, dried fruit especially apricots, eggs, raw oysters, wheat germs, almonds, beans, lima beans and meat are foods high in iron.

One last word about minerals, the skin is the largest organ on or in our bodies. You can absorb more chlorine, salt and toxic chemicals from 24 normal baths or showers than you can ingesting them over a 5 year period. A 150 lb. person can gain 3 lbs. of weight in a 20 minute bath or shower. So if you are conscientious of what you put into your body you should be just as conscientious as to what you put on your body or into your bath water.

A little known additive called Tyramine is found in sharp cheeses and Chianti red wine. This has been known to cause headaches with rapid rises in blood pressure in people taking the drug Monoamine Oxidase. This drug is used for psychiatric disorders such as depression, insomnia, and in certain phobic anxiety states, plus it lowers blood pressures. However, toxicity in this drug is relatively great and an added hazard to looking our best.

Generally substances such as caffeine, nicotine, alcohol, food additives and prescription drugs can rob our energy and adversely affect our bodies. Coffee is a major source of Cadmium, a toxic mineral which has been linked to heart disease and high blood pressure. Heavy coffee and tea drinkers inhibit the bodies ability to absorb iron. And Alcoholics are usually deficient in Magnesium and Potassium. All of this throws off body balance and causes stress.

When people say it's too difficult to give up what they enjoy, then I believe in compromise. Try cutting down on known stress factors. No need to put both mental and physical stress on the body by quitting cold turkey unless you can handle it. But do minimize these products and try substituting herb teas for regular and imitation coffee in place of the usual nerve stimulator even if you only replace one cup a day. In other words, if you need to drink regular teas and coffees then have one cup of regular and one of something else. The body can usually handle that much without too many problems. By the way, the chemicals they use to decaffinate coffee are not any better for you than regular coffee. Ralph Nader researchers found out that a chemical used in some ground and instant decaffinated coffee has produced a "frighteningly high" incidence of cancer in test animals and should be banned — but isn't. The chemical, trichlorethylene, TCE, is used to remove caffeine but traces of it remain in the coffee and can even be inhaled from the coffee fumes. Another study performed by the Cancer Institute involved mice fed both high and low doses of TCE. Even in the low dose group 30 percent developed liver cancer. Personally I'd rather take my chances with regular coffee. But as I have said, cut down and perhaps you will find you don't mind skipping a day or two between usage. Overdoing what we enjoy is a problem many of us have but when we overdo the body cannot detoxity itself fast enough to prevent damage. Water process decaf coffee is now available.

If a person consumes more than two alcoholic drinks at a sitting then the liver has difficulty taking out the harmful ingredients before the body sustains damage in some area. Another problem with "modern" liquor as with so many of our food and drinks today is that it is highly processed and chemically treated so that practically all the vitamin and mineral content is lost.

However, take heart, it isn't only the products we seem to enjoy that cause body stress. Excessive amounts of cabbage, turnips, rutabagas, brussel sprouts and broccoli can reduce the thyroid gland's ability to regulate body functions such as fat metabolism and energy production. People who have eaten large amounts of cabbage for long periods have been known to develop goiters. Other natural foods that might have toxicity if used to excess are beets, parsley, rhubarb, swiss chard, cocoa, celery and spinach. They all contain a food substance called oxalates and too much oxalates will reduce calcium absorption. When the body has a reduction in calcium, teeth will decay more readily, bones become brittle, nails split, hair dries out and the skin wrinkles more rapidly than normal because of bone shrinkage. But since most people are not overly fond of vegetables the chances of overeating them are rather small.

Seeds, beans, corn, grains, potatoes and soybeans contain phytates and in excess they may inhibit the absorption of minerals and iron. Cooking these foods even very little destroys the phytates, also sprouting seeds and grains destroys phytates.

Raw egg white has a substance called avidin that prevents the absorption of biotin, biotin is essential for metabolism of fats and proteins and is part of the B-Complex family, but boiling eggs for as little as twenty seconds eliminates this problem. Foods known to be high in biotin are nuts, fruits,

Brewer's Yeast, brown rice, egg yolk, and milk. Biotin is also reputed to help keep your hair its natural color.

It's important that the body be helped in its metabolism because metabolism, as previously stated, is the sum of the chemical changes in living organisms and cells by which food is converted into living protoplasm, and by which protoplasm is used and broken down into simpler compounds and waste by liberation of energy. Anyone who looks like they are depleted of energy also looks old just through body language. It is not just junk foods that cause body stress and premature aging.

But, whole fresh foods in the right amounts can keep us from rapid aging. Nutrition expert the late Dr. Paavo Airola, said a diet of raw whole unprocessed natural food is rich in enzymes and enzymes are the powerful catalysts which direct and control all chemical reactions and life processes including digestion and assimilation.

The most important thing to remember is that your diet needs are constantly changing from day to day. Your body could be perfectly fine today and listless tomorrow depending on many causes, i.e., diet, stress, emotions, exercise or lack of, and mental attitude.

Both men and women go through a "change of life" sometime between 40 to 44 on an average. With women the change is more physically evident with the cessation of menses. But with men the physical changes do bring physical and emotional stress and when men try to act like nothing is happening they often suffer from such varied ailments as depression, degenerative diseases, heart attacks and what is known as "second childhood" behavior that seems rather silly for their age.

As the essential adrenal hormones in our bodies start to decline, complaints of arthritis, bursitis, colitis, nephritis and all kinds of various allergies arise. That's when TV commercials tell us what to take to cover up the pain but they don't tell us what to take to really rid the body of the problem. To me, that's like covering garbage, you may hide it but it still stinks.

The body's *Dis-Ease* can be fought in a number of natural ways. An excellent way to help the body fight off aches and pains is by simply eating onions and garlic at least once a week. When I started doing this I got amazing results. Joint aches that I had grown accustomed to disappeared after a few weeks of usage. Of course, the best time to do this is when you know you'll be home alone or at least when you know you're not going to be communicating passionately with someone else. Although as mentioned before now they do have odorless garlic capsules and tablets. Also garlic tablets with parsley are available at some health food stores.

If you have a tendency toward anemia do not eat raw garlic. Take Kyolic aged garlic extract.

When I discovered the odorles garlic product called Kyolic, I was intrigued because like most people the odor of garlic was a turn off so I investigated further to find out if odorless is just as beneficial as regular garlic and to my delight I found it is.

The whole garlic bulb contains natural antibiotics, anti-fungual, antibacterial and anti-oxidants. It stimulates digestive juices, is an excellent diuretic and anti-clotting agent. It also contains over 36 theraputic sulfur compounds, 3 enzymes and a bit of Vitamins A, C, E, Thiamine, Riboflavin and Niacin. It has minute amounts of iodine, iron, calcium, maganese and potassium. Garlic is rich in sulfur, a body balancer helping to regulate the hormones and enzymes it takes to keep us well. The odor of garlic is produced when a sulfur Amino Acid called Alliin combines with an enzyme called Allinase when garlic is cut or crushed. They combine to create 18 odor causing compounds including allicin. Not only is raw garlic offensive but in large quantities allicin can destroy the membranes of red blood cells and inflame the gastrointestinal tract. Too much of this could cause anemia and stomach problems. That's why raw garlic is not recommended for people with ulcers, colitis or irritable bowel syndrome. Fortunately, back in 1954, Dr. Eugene Schnell, former supervisor of Japanese pharmaceutical regulations for the United States Government, got together with a Japanese banker named Mangi Wakunaga to perfect a natural cold aging odorless garlic (Kyolic) to act as a potent immune enhancer. In other words have Kyolic stimulate the body's own defense mechanism to protect itself.

The latest research on garlic's medicinal value now lies in the conversion of allicin to more beneficial sulphur compounds. One such compound called Diallysulfide has been found to be beneficial in colon cancer treatment. Ajoene is another compound found in garlic and has shown to be beneficial inhibiting blood platelet aggregation. Studies conducted in the Wakunaga Laboratories and repeated in Japanese hospitals showed that Kyolic helps rid the body of smog; the ozone and photochemical pollution caused by nitrous oxides; heavy metal poisoning from lead, mercury and copper; and food and water contaminated by chemicals, pesticides, waste fluids and food additives such as sodium cyclamates.

Research done at Kunamoto University by toxicology professor, Dr. Satosi Kitahara showed that Kyolic helps prevents heart disease and atherosclerosis by cutting cholesterol levels in the blood and it is effective against gastrointestinal disorders, hypoglycemia, hemorrhoids, diabetes, anemia and dysentery. Garlic reduces the stickiness of platelets, increases the fibrinolytic or anticlotting activity and elevates the beneficial HDL's and fights germs that cause pneumonia, tuberculosis, diptheria, typhus and the common cold. One of the principle difference between raw garlic and Kyolic (other than odor) is this fact: raw garlic is a strong oxidizer. Kyolic acts as anti-oxidant. The anti-oxidants are essential for activating the bodies own immune responses to fight cell destruction.

The problem is where can one find the right soil in todays polluted world? Mr. Wakunaga found it in the northernmost part of Japan's four main islands, Hokkaido. There he had his workers plough fields and compost for four years before growing a single clove of garlic. Then he hired agriculture school graduates to supervise the cultivation from start to finish. The garlic in Kyolic is grown organically. Commercially grown garlic in the United States is treated with formaldehyde, herbicides are used for weed control, and commercial fertilizers high in nitrates are added to the soil. No crop rotation is used. Wakunaga believes that good health comes from the soil. Wakunaga treats their soil with respect not chemicals.

The philosophy at Wakunaga is dedicated to improving the health and welfare of people all over the world. Their motto is: As important as Kyolic is — it is just one spoke in the wheel of optimum health. Life style and diet are just as important as any food supplement. Preventive medicine is the best medicine — and the best healer of all is the body's own immune system.

Garlic stimulates the immune system helping to prevent not only cancer and heart disease but herpes and even AIDS. A staff physician, Dr. Tariq Abdullah at the Akbar Clinic and Research Institute in Panama City, Fla. says his research involved three groups of volunteers. One group ate a small amount of raw garlic, another took Kyolic garlic capsules and the third took no garlic. The cells taken from the group that ate the raw garlic killed 138% more cancer cells than those from the group that ate no garlic. And "killer" cells taken from the group that ate the Kyolic garlic capsules destroyed 159% more tumor cells than cells taken from the non-garlic group. Dr. Abdullah says he uses Kyolic garlic because it is the only commercial garlic preparation which is processed by cold rather than by heat. Heating or cooking garlic destroys many of garlic's therapeutic compounds.

It takes nearly two years (exactly 20 months) to produce Kyolic odorless garlic because it is done naturally.

A nutritional consultant and dear friend of mine in Los Angeles, Sally Kelly, told me that she uses and recommends Kyolic liquid garlic for ear aches. She runs hot water over the dropper and fills it half full of liquid Kyolic and puts it into the sore ear. Sally said sometimes when she takes a plane trip she will get off with an earache but as soon as she puts Kyolic liquid in her ear the pain disappears within minutes. Sally is a great believer in homeopathic remedies and recommends Arnica for bruising and pain from injuries not only as tablets but as liquid that can be rubbed on the sore spot.

Among her other favorites are Icthammol ointment for relieving the pain of ingrown toenails and splinters under the skin. Ichthammol helps bring the injury out while it relieves the pain.

For smoggy days she recommends a homepathic remedy called Petroleum and this is also helpful for the irritated eyes of people who wear contact lenses. If you have broken bones, Symphitiam, it's made from Comfrey Root and seems to help bones mend faster.

Now for all of us who love animals an interesting news release came from a leading northern California veterinarian, Dr. Gloria Dodd of Danville, Calif. Dr. Dodd is the founder and former President of the California Holistic Veterinarian Medical Association. She calls herself an "Evangelistic Born-Again Veterinarian." Her latest project is the development of an animal First-Aid Kit with a handbook illustrating 33 different emergency problems. It includes everything from instructions on how to make a temporary splint out of rolled newspapers to a vial of honey bee extract to counteract bee sting or other venemous insect bites. The collection of homeopathic remedies includes no drugs — that would be too dangerous. These herbs are identified by Dr. Dodd for their usefulness in injury or illness.

The Animal First-Aid Emergency Kit book and tapes are available by writing to Dr. Dodd at 857 El Pintado Rd., Danville, CA 94526 or you may phone (415) 837-7759, for further information.

Dr. Dodd reports that additives in dog and cat food can cause a variety of reactions in pets including skin rashes, loss of coat lustre, diabetes, digestive disturbances and even epileptic seizures and death. Dr. Dodd reports that many commercial pet foods contain insecticides, herbicides, cortisone, hormones and heavy metals such as aluminum but with treatments of Kyolic these toxic substances could be eliminated naturally. Kyolic helped to break down the toxins without upsetting the animals delicate digestive system. Because the garlic odor has been removed from Kyolic the capsules and liquid extract can be easily mixed with food. Dr. Dodd reported that dogs were dying of the immune deficiency syndrome. There was nothing Vets could do about it but now they are not only saving pets lives they are also improving ailments like heart disease, arthritis and breath odor with the continuous use of Kyolic.

Garlic seems to inhibit clumping of lymphocytes. Lymphocytes clumping allows viruses to pass from one lymphocyte to the other as the viruses pass around the body. Many of the sulfur containing compounds in garlic are free radical scavengers and anti-oxidants and these compounds protect people and pets from the free radical damage caused by the innumerable food additives.

A little known fact is 6% of the dry weight of garlic is made of bioflavanoids (Quecitin and cyanidin). Bioflavanoids have anti-viral, anti-inflamatory and anti-oxidant properties. Not only this but the bioflavanoids deaggregate blood cells which mean they don't clot and the blood flows easily.

Immunoligist, Benjamin Lau, M.D., Ph.D., Professor of Microbiology, School of Medicine, Loma Linda University, has reported the cure of a mouse tumor with C. Parvum Vaccine with Kyolic garlic extract. The breakthrough was published in the September '86 issue of the Journal of Urology. Five consecutive treatments with the Kyolic extract stopped the growth of cancer, while the same number of treatments with the orthodox vaccine reduced the growth about 50%. Dr. Lau cautions that success in animals should not be translated directly to success for humans. Dr. Lau points out that it appears that the Kyolic inactivated the sulfhydral compounds in the tumor cells and then elicited the NK (Natural Killer) cells leading to the destruction of the tumor cells.

More recently Dr. Lau used Kyolic garlic liquid extract to treat patients with elevated serum cholesterol and triglycerides. Dr. Lau found not only Kyolic lowered these levels but it raised high density lipoprotein. Such changes are highly beneficial to the cardiovascular system. (Nutrition Research Vol. 7, Page 139). Another result of Dr. Lau's study is interesting to note. Kyolic appears to be *selective* in that it did not significantly influence the levels of cholesterol and triglycerides in subjects whose initial cholesterol levels were relatively low, but produced positive reductions in those with initially high levels of cholesterol.

Dr. Lau's book, "Garlic for Health" got rave

reviews on Paul Harvey's national radio show. This book is must reading for everyone.

Finally, garlic has important value not only to scientists, but to athletes, as well. It is an excellent stamina food supplement.

Dozens of well-known athletes, such as Ray Beaulieu, two-time Mr. Canada; use garlic regularly. Roger Marshall, the alpinist currently ranked second in the world uses Kyolic odorless garlic extract to improve his oxygen utilization and circulatory capacity at high altitudes. Tom Magee of Canada is the only man to win the title of strongest man in the world 3 years in a row. Tom takes Kyolic everyday. He says it's indispensable.

No other vegetable has ever received so much praise and attention from researchers and physicians around the world. Garlic is used to fight diseases, enrich diets, improve health and most important — prolong life.

HEALTH FACTS

Some people have no digestion problems when eating onions and garlic raw but others find slight cooking makes them palatable. As stated, onions and garlic are natural germ fighters having antibiotic and anti-histamine properties and they also help fight a build-up of cholesterol. Some nutritionists say they prevent hair loss.

If you eat at least one green salad a day you are probably getting enough chlorophyll and if you eat plain unsugared yogurt you are getting acidophilus (that's the friendly bacteria). If you hate yogurt, acidophilus is available in liquid, tablets or capsule form. A good nutritional doctor will always prescribe acidophilus after the use of antibiotics because the antibiotics can't tell good bacteria from bad so all bacteria gets destroyed. The good bacteria should be helped to return as quickly as possible. Acidophilus has also been helpful in the treatment of acne and other skin problems.

Everyone has bad breath at one time or another but if you want to eliminate it don't put some candy confection in your mouth, take a tablespoon of liquid acidophilus and a tablespoon of liquid chlorophyll. Your teeth and your body will thank you for it. Having good solid teeth is important to delaying wrinkles because when you start losing teeth the face begins to sag. If you've ever seen anyone who wears false teeth when they're not wearing them then that picture is worth a thousand words.

So even if a tooth dies, I recommend trying root canal work and leaving the tooth in place. Any reputable dentist will always try to save your own teeth first before recommending the store bought kind.

I'd like to mention a skin problem that had the spotlight before AIDS — Herpes Simplex. This is a viral skin infection characterized by a cluster of small blisters of watery vesicles on the skin or mucus membranes. This viral problem seems to be part of the price people pay for turning from social intercourse to sexual intercourse on a grand scale. This tiny microscope virus has done more to convince people of their errant ways than all the fire and brimstone preachers in the world. The herpes lesions are commonly called cold sores or fever blisters and most often occur on the lips and face but occasionally on the genitals, trunk, buttocks and hands. When a lesion it is often accompanied by a tingling and burning in the skin area which becomes red and covered with vesicles. These vesicles break and form a crust and the skin appears normal in 6 to 10 days unless there has been a secondary infection.

So far science has not found a cure for this virus and the lesions may reappear at the same site for many years and may be precipitated by sunburn, upper-respiratory and gastro-intestinal infections, fevers, emotional stress, anxiety or when you are generally run down and exhausted. Naturally all these irritations can make the skin appear older.

But take heart, a multicentered dermatology study has found something that appears to suppress the clinical manifestations (cutaneous lesions) of herpes virus infection. Patients (45) with frequently recurring herpes infection were given between 312 to 1200 mg. of Lysine daily in single or multiple doses. The Clinical results demonstrated a beneficial effect from supplementary lysine in accelerating recovery from herpes simplex infection and suppressing recurrence. Lysine is a basic amino acid produced chiefly from proteins and is essential to nutrition. Anyone who has this problem should ask their doctor about this.

PINES WHEAT GRASS

All life depends on the sun. Sunlight activates the green chlorophyll in plants to generate energy for the plants.

A fine source of chlorophyll is Pines Wheat Grass. Chlorophyll has a strong attraction for oxygen and carries the oxygen wherever it goes in the body. Many germs that invade the human body prefer to grow in tissues where there is a poor supply of oxygen. Japanese researchers have demonstrated the juice of green plants inhibit chromosome damage, which is one of the links in the chain of events leading to cancer.

Pines Wheat grass comes in powder, tablets, and frozen juice. Best of all Pines Wheat Grass is organically grown in rich mineral soil in Laurence, Kansas. Pines Wheat Grass is rich in amino acids, beta-carotene, minerals and enzymes. Pines Wheat Grass is dehydrated at room temperature and is an excellent source of concentrated chlorophyll.

Dr. Krebs the discoverer of Laetrile (Vitamin B-17) has identified Wheat Grass as a good source of B-17.

Pines Wheat Grass tablets swell up to 12 times their size when wet and are a good source of fiber. In fact it has twice as much fiber as bran, without the irritation.

Fresh wheat grass juice can be obtained at most health food stores or you can learn to harvest this source of chlorophyll with a minimum of work in your home.

All the research done on wheat grass has been done on the dehydrated not the fresh juice. Five tablets of dehydrated wheat grass supply the nutritional equivalent of a half cup of finely chopped fresh kale or collards.

Did you know that laboratories have found Pines wheat grass to be one of the best foods to grow experimental samples of the beneficial bacteria needed by the human digestive tract!

Wheat grass needs to grow slowly during the cold weather of winter and early spring in climates like Kansas. It must be harvested during a 4 day period in April to obtain the high levels of nutrients.

Wheat grass' optimum concentration of vitamins, minerals and chlorophyll is only obtained by growing the wheat grass for at least 60 days in fresh air, sunlight, and cold temperature.

The best of land and sea chlorophyll is now obtainable in a tasty and nutritious drink. The product is called Kyo-Green and is available in health food stores. It is an excellent immune booster.

Kyo-Green contains the juice powder of organic wheat and barley grass, broken cell chlorella, kelp and brown rice. Kyo-Green mixes easily and is sodium free.

ALUMINUM

The U.S. government and food and drug manufacturers are equal partners in determining the aluminum contents of their products. We receive a complex double message from the FDA, who warn us of toxic dangers while approving chemical additives to food, water processing plants, medical and skin care products. Associated pharmacologists and toxicologists estimate the average human ingests 22 to 100 milligrams of aluminum each day and as much as 25 percent may remain in the body.

Aluminum powders repel moisture and bugs, lengthening market shelf life of more foods than most of us could ever imagine. This includes Aunt Jemima, Duncan Hines, Jeno's Pizza, flour, baking powder, breads, processed cheese. Read the package labels.

Aluminum is the major buffering agent for

aspirin. But accumulative amounts may be deforming to brain cells, creating the symptoms of Alzheimer' disease. The FDA has instructed aspirin makers to cease recommending the drug as a heart medication. (Please note: Aspirin companies do not always list their ingredients on the outside packaging.)

Deodorants, skin creams, vaginal hygiene powders, antacids, aspirin, commercial foods and public drinking water may contain one or more of the following: alumina, aluminum glycinate, aluminum zirconium, sodium aluminum phosphate, aluminum hyroxide or titanium.

This information is important to people who are experiencing difficulties in medical diagnosis. American Health Magazine (October 1963) physicians report a possibility that a certain percentage of the population retains aluminum and other toxic metals in the tissues similar to allergy-prone individuals. (This could translate to a number of mental and depression symptoms that may be eliminated if reversed in early stages of development.)

Until the arrival of the Alzheimer's age, no one thought aluminum to be dangerous. Expedient use of a remarkable metal has created a problem of overuse. If indeed, human ingestion of metal pollutants is the cause of brain disease, then Alzheimer is preventable and curable. But it means we must change our style of life. We are responsible for how we care. We are responsible for the people we elect to represent us on important issues. And we are responsible for the products we choose to buy.

JUICERS

No kitchen should ever be without an electric juice extractor! What better way to get a fresh supply of nature's vitamins, minerals and enzymes. All are quickly assimilated by the body for energy and vigor.

The benefits of superior nutrition are there for all including those persons with chewing and digestion problems. Juices are instant energy boosters.

Reward yourself and your family with a Juice Extractor and get the most out of what comes naturally.

The Juice Extractor we would never be without is the Olympic Juicer. It's one of the prized possessions in my kitchen arsenal.

The Olympic Juicer is manufactured in the United States, has precise balancing, the very best engineering, a smooth and quiet operation and is easy to use and clean. From start to finish the juice will only contact surgical stainless steel.

Best of all the Olympic Juicer comes with an incredible 10 year unconditional guarantee.

The Olympic Juicer is manufactured by Olympic Products, Inc., P.O. Box 4523, Harrisburg, PA 17111 — Phone No. (717) 652-8760 or 1 (800) 633-3401.

CHAPTER 8
Homeopathy

Many sciences of health care have evolved over the thousands of years that humans have been on planet earth. Many of these sciences have provided us with valuable tools for diagnosis and treatment of ill health. In fact, what is known as modern medicine has only been around less than 100 years, while the ancient Chinese and Indian systems are about 6,000 years old.

The principles of homeopathy have existed for approximately 3000 years compared to approximately 40 years of modern drugs. Homeopathy comes from two Greek words, "Homeo" and "pathos" meaning a similar suffering. It is similar to immunization. And is described as "like curing like." In India it is still the health care of 350 million people. In the West homeopathy was re-discovered in the

17th Century by Dr. Samuel Hahnemann in Germany.

As we entered the 20th Century, about 25% of the physicians in America were homeopaths but less than 25 years later the allopaths in America formed the American Medical Assn. and homeopathy fell behind as chemical drugs took over.

However, fortunately there is now a new interest in the natural curing energies of this science. So now there is much to draw upon in our search for health and many of the available tools are easily understood by the average person seeking good health.

Since this book is about rejuvenation, I became fascinated in the Oriental system of medicine whereby they use facial lines to diagnose the state of body health. From the books, "Healing Ourselves" by Naboru Muramoti and "Oriental Diagnosis" by Michio Kushi, I learned which lines indicate which body problems.

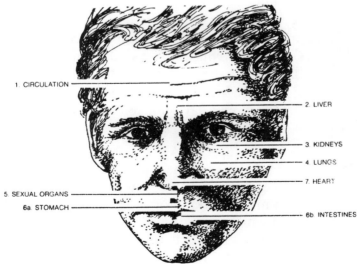

This facial line chart reflects Oriental diagnostic methods and is only meant to be a guide to your health. Always remember that diagnosis is an art as well as a science and requires knowledge, practice and skill. If there is any doubt about your state of health contact a professional.

PROSTAGLANDINS

Every living cell in the human body has a liquid coating which is made up of fats. These fats come from the food we eat. An important function of fats in the body is to balance a class of chemicals called prostaglandins.

Prostaglandins regulate the body's inflamatory response and these prostagladins are made from the essential fatty acids from the food we eat.

Essential fatty acids come from beans and seeds. The only substantial source of GLA is the seed oil from the evening primrose plant. The yellow flower it produces twines up the stem and dies after a single evening — hence it's name. The reason for this plant's recent rise to the height of medical stardom lies in the contents of these seeds. Reports from Europe showed it to be quite successful in Pre-Menstrual Tension (PMS), Multiple Scleroses (MS), heart disease, eczema, alcoholism, and even weight loss cases.

Large deposits of EFA are found in the thymus. When the EFA stores in the body are low — there is an imbalance in the immune system. One of the critical EFA's in the making of prostaglandins is cis-linoleic acid which is converted to gamma-linolenic acid (GLA). Two products that I recommend for a superior source of Primrose Oil are Effamol and Gama Oil.

BACK FLOWER REMEDIES

Ah, flowers! Flowers are aesthetically pleasing to the senses and that is why we enjoy looking at them but it wasn't until I discovered the Bach flower remedies that I really got into the study of flowers.

It was then that I found out what FLOWER POWER really means. At a time when I was deeply distressed by personal misfortune and by the misfortune of a friend, into my life walked Leslie Kaslof and brought "RESCUE REMEDY," a fast first aid for emotional distress.

I took four drops of this Rescue Remedy under my tongue and within minutes I felt calmer. Now some might say it was psychological, that the mere suggestion of a name like Rescue Remedy would help to make me feel better. OK, if that is the case, then Great, because my motto has always been:

WHATEVER WORKS!

Homeopathic remedies should help to strengthen, heal and energize the body. The main idea is to give nature a chance to work her curative powers. Many times when people are having emotional problems the Bach flower remedies are very helpful in calming the nerves, relieving anxiety and fear, alleviating depression and balancing out feelings of guilt or lack of confidence.

However, because it is my nature, I had to further investigate these flowers remedies. I enrolled for a weekend seminar on Bach Flower Remedies and there I listened to Leslie and bought some books on the subject. I also bought all the remedies and when I'm emotionally distressed I mix myself a little flower power. During the seminar Mr. Kaslof said, "The main reason for the failure of modern medical science is they deal with results and not causes." He recommended reading, "THE BACH FLOWER REMEDIES" which includes, "Heal Thyself" and "The Twelve Healers" by Edward Bach, M.D. plus "The Bach Remedies Repertory" by F.J. Wheeler, M.D. and I would like to quote a small section from the book which I totally agree with:

"Every time a person thinks negative or depressing thoughts, it chips away their health because the thymus stops working for that moment.

That is why I am against most psychotherapy; because it focuses on the negative and the thymus is continually being pounded. A healthy thymus is associated with love, joy, youth and enthusiasm.

Hate and envy seem to rob the body and all the organs of energy, the kind of energy that is associated with acupuncture. The gland that seems to be particularly affected by hate and envy is the thymus. As long as the patient has an underactive thymus gland, none of the immune systems will work properly."

The thymus gland structure is largely lymphoid tissue that functions in cell-mediated immunity by being the site where T-cells develop. Lately T-cells have been very prominent in the news as one of the immune systems defenses against AIDS.

Moral: Be kind to yourself by being kind to your neighbor. Let love live again and it will help you to stay well.

Some cancer researchers are applying positive thinking to remove serious illness. They teach cancer patients to imagine their healthy white blood cells are devouring tumors.

The point I'm trying to make is that because we do have problems that weigh heavily on us emotionally, we need to find ways to help us get through emotional distress.

Dr. Bach distilled the essence of certain flowers in an effort to relieve emotional distress without using chemical drugs that might have adverse side effects. Long before any of his colleagues accepted it, he believed that our fears and anxieties open the pathway to the invasion of illness. So in order to help people better cope with fear, uncertainty, loneliness, anxiety and despair he put together 38 remedies.

Now when I look at the visual beauty of such flowers as Impatience, Honeysuckle and Wild Rose I think how nice that these lovely flowers help us inside and out. Just as the name implies, Impatience helps people who are always rushing and impatient, Honeysuckle is given to those who live too much in the past and Wild Rose is used for those who are resigned to all that happens with apathy.

Personally, I am still studying and experimenting with these remedies because much of life is a continuous learning experience.

By the year 2000 there will be almost 40 million people who are 65 or older and we are now living in an era that has been termed the "Graying of America." Wouldn't it be nice if we could help each other to lead happy, healthy and useful lives right up to the moment we leave this planet and start our next journey.

Unfortunately we live in a drug culture at the present time and it is taking its toll, not only in more physical disabilities but also in more homicides and suicides. We can only hope and pray that more people will come to realize how really precious their bodies are and with this awareness will come the ability to be more discerning about what they use on or put into those bodies.

SALT

Salt is in all packaged, processed and fast foods unless otherwise stated on the label. The problem with most salt free foods is they taste bland so unless you have a problem with high blood pressure then I would say don't worry about salt in your diet but DO NOT add it to your food.

If you do have to buy salt free foods you can add taste with all kinds of different herbs and spices that are offered at health food stores or health food sections of super markets.

A good salt substitute for Popcorn is natural yeast with selenium and/or Dr. Bronner's balanced mineral seasoning. If you don't have a problem with high blood pressure then melt lightly salted raw butter over the popcorn.

Some people with high blood pressure have lowered the pressure by simply cleaning their colons with high fiber foods, garlic or special colon cleanser products. Others have done this with enemas or colonics. Internal cleansing often helps to balance the body.

I do not believe in chemical salt substitutes or for that matter chemical sugar substitutes. The body will metabolize salt and sugar but chemicals are not metabolized and cause the body stress. Body stress of any kind can break down the immune system.

Be very careful of dairy substitute foods they are often loaded with chemicals, salt and fats.

CELL SALTS

Cell salts are another special supplement. The basis of biochemistry was discovered over a hundred years ago when Rudolph Virchow, a scientist, realized that the human body is composed of an enormous number of tiny, living cells, infinitesimal but perfectly balanced with three classes of materials: Water, Organic Materials and Inorganic Substances.

Water and organic materials such as sugar, albuminous and fatty matter make up the greater portion, but inorganic mineral elements are vital active workers which utilize the organic substances in building the millions of cells of which the body is composed. The life of our cells is short, they are constantly breaking down and being replaced by new ones and the necessary material for this rebuilding is supplied by the bloodstream. There are 12 Cell Salts or tissue salts in our bodies. Dr. W. Schuessler, a physiological chemist and physicist, originated the "Biochemic System of Medicine" and coined the word "Biochemistry." The 12 Cell Salts are Calcium Sulphate, Phosphate of Iron, Potassium Chloride, Potassium Phosphate, Potassium Sulphate, Magnesium Phosphate, Sodium Chloride, Sodium Phosphate, Sodium Sulphate, Silica, Calcium Fluoride and Calcium Phosphate. The body must have a balance of all these to run efficiently.

Disturbed metabolism is undoubtedly one of the major causes of accelerated aging. Metabolism is the process by which the body converts food into living tissue. Metabolism encompasses digestion, assimilation, tissue renovation and the provision of body heat and energy. Studies have shown that in middle age the tendency to disturbances in metabolism and to tissue salt deficiences is increased. The only way to know if your body metabolism is working efficiently is to listen to your own body. If it aches and pains it is telling you something is wrong. Pay attention to yourself first because without you there is nothing. When you think about that, you will realize that truer words were never spoken. So become an assistant to your doctor and you will never get better care.

If you need supplements to help your body work more efficiently then find what is best for you. In some cases all the supplements are needed: vitamins, minerals, herbs and cell salts plus special dietary foods but in other cases none are necessary. I would consult with a nutritionally minded medical doctor before experimenting with supplements.

Digestive problems are quite common these days usually because we gulp our food down in haste or because we eat when we are nervous or not really hungry. Antacids only cover up the problem. I would recommend taking a digestive enzyme pill as an aid to helping the stomach fluids break down our food into the basic body building nutrients we need. Digestive enzymes usually contain at least one or more of the following ingredients: Pancreatin, Glutamic Acid, Hydrochloride, Ox Bile Extract, Pepsin,

Papain and Duodenum. The green leaves of Alfalfa have 8 necessary enzymes. Alfalfa contains Vitamins A, E, B6, K, D, U and some phosphorus and lime. It also helps the body in elimination.

Included in my diet to help digestion are Kyodophilus, Kyo-green, Kyolic formula 102, liquid chlorophyll, wheat germ, kelp, yeast and, if I have heartburn, a tablespoon of Aloe Vera Gel. Aloe Vera is extracted from a cactus looking plant. More on Aloe Vera later.

The Cell Salts recommended for digestion are Sodium and Calcium Phosphate. Calcium Fluoride gives the tissues the quality of elasticity. But the best way to learn if you need Cell Salts is to read Dr. W. Schuessler's Biochemic Handbook."

About once every two or three months I might make a sea salt and Epsom salt paste and wash my face and neck with it. This helps to shed dead skin and stimulate circulation. But, again, one must really know their own skin. Some people are too sensitive for this. However, body salt rubs are often given at health spas in the belief that they remove dead skin and body toxins.

Now as stated Cell Salts are an entirely different salt from any Epsom, Sea or regular table salt and I would like to give a more detailed review of them now.

Cell Salts are tissue salts inside our bodies. The human body is composed of trillions of tiny cells, each of which is a complete living unit. These cells differ in composition according to the type of tissue they help to form.

The cells forming bone are different from those

forming skin or nerve tissue. The material from which these cells are maintained comes or should come from our own food. It is of 2 kinds, organic and inorganic. Organic materials are albumin, fibrin, sugar and fats. The inorganic materials are water and certain minerals, known as mineral or tissue cell salts.

The term, Biochemistry, means the chemistry of life. The biochemistry of the body is the trillions of cells that work within it. Our bodies are born with the right amount of cell salts but as we get older they start to deplete and the work of repairing and replacing should be done by the food we eat. That used to be the case when we had foods that were not chemically sprayed and processed to the point where nutrition is at a minimum. Fortunately, today when we find we have a deficiency in one of these salts we can supplement them.

There are 12 tissue salts or cell salts in the body that have been identified and labeled. Actually there are traces of many more but Dr. W. H. Schuesssler (1821 to 1898) was the first to rediscover these cell salts in modern times.

Since humans are a microcosm in the macrocosm it is possible that there are traces of every mineral found upon this planet in our bodies. Biochemistry is an ancient Sanskrit science but I first discovered Cell Salts when an Astrologer, Alice Lane, did my astrological chart and told me that according to my chart I needed certain cell salts. She said the position and aspects of the moon and major planets will show what minerals a person is likely to be deficient in. That intrigued me enough to find out more about the basic science of cell salts.

At that time I was having a problem with paper thin cracks in my facial skin that wouldn't seem to heal. I had tried creams and lotions and salves to no avail. When I read a pamphlet on cells salts I found that Calcium Fluoride is present in the surface of bones, in the enamel of teeth, and in the elastic fibers of the skin, muscular tissue and blood vessels. I went to my local health food store, bought some and began taking it. Within 2 days my skin cracks healed. Of course, then I was hooked. I had to study about all 12 cells salts to find out what they did in the body and then I decided to take a combination of all 12, which I do periodically when I feel I need it and an extra supplement of one particular salt if I have a problem.

THE 12 CELL SALTS

CALCIUM FLUORIDE

Gives tissue elasticity. If you have a relaxed condition of veins, arteries, piles, sluggish circulation, a tendency to cracks in the skin, notably in the palms, between the toes and on the face then Calcium Fluoride is beneficial.

CALCIUM PHOSPATE

Promotes healthy cellular activity and restores tone to a weakened organ or tissue, a condition that often happens after pregnancy or a large amount of weight gain.

CALCIUM SULPHATE

A blood purifier and healer. Found in the liver where it helps in removal of waste from the blood stream and has a cleansing and purifying influence throughout the system.

FERRUM PHOSPHATE

Also called Phospate of Iron, is an oxygen carrier. It takes up oxygen from the air and carries it into the blood stream to all parts of the body furnishing the vital force that sustains life.

POTASSIUM CHLORIDE

Also known as Kali Mur, is a remedy for sluggish conditions. It is important to digestion. A deficiency causes catarrh and mucous discharges.

POTASIUM PHOSPHATE

Also called Kali Phosphate is a nerve nutrient. It helps maintain a happy contented disposition. It is a remedy for lowered vitality, depression, weariness and a general lack of pep. A condition that happens periodically to everyone.

POTASSIUM SULPHATE

Also called Kali Sulphate, works in conjunction with Iron Phosphate as an oxygen carrier. It assists in the exchange of oxygen from the blood stream to the tissue cells. Internal breathing of the tissues depends upon this cell salt. External breathing is the function of Iron Phosphate. Eruptions on the skin and scalp, with scaling and intestinal disorders call for this salt.

MAGNESIUM PHOSPHATE

Also called Mag. Phos., is important to muscular tissue and rhythmic movement. Helps relieve pain from cramps and spasms, menstrual stomach cramps and flatulence.

SODIUM CHLORIDE

Maintains a proper degree of moisture throughout the body. It helps produce hydrochloric acid which aids digestion. Two thirds of the body is composed of water and too little or too much can have a direct effect on the skin.

SODIUM PHOSPHATE

Also known as Nat. Phos., helps balance acid in the blood. A deficiency could cause Uric Acid to form salts which become deposited around the joints and tissues giving stiffness and swelling.

SODIUM SULPHATE

Also called Nat. Sulph., helps keep the liver functioning with a supply of bile. There are chemical exchanges constantly taking place in the tissue cells and this salt helps remove the poisons from the fluids.

SILICA

Also known as Silicic Oxide, is a constituent of the blood, hair, skin, nails and bone surfaces. It is a cleanser and eliminator in helping the body throw off non-functional organic matter. It is an insulator for the nerves. Silica acts upon the organic substances of the body; i.e. bones, joints, glands and skin and can be used where there is pus formations like pimples, abscesses, boils and styes. Often it helps brittle nails and lifeless hair.

CHAPTER 9

Water

Alcohol is out! Water is in! In fact one of the most profitable bars in Beverly Hills is now a water bar. Water is big business. People who are interested in their health know that the type of water they drink can add or detract from it.

Of course, basic to our nutrition is the water we drink. Water makes up over 80 percent of our body. The brain contains 74.5 percent, bones 22 percent, muscle 75.6 percent, kidney 82.7 percent and blood 83 percent.

Over 95 million Americans drink Fluoridated water. Some think it is good for them, others don't have a choice because it was added to their drinking water by city government. Now, however, increasing numbers of researchers and scientists believe that Sodium Fluoride (which is a rat poison in large doses) and which is added to public water supplies to prevent tooth decay actually causes allergies, arthritic like pains in the joints, brittle bones, nervousness and even cancer, and recently it is believed to predispose people to AIDS. They have also discovered that people with diabetes, kidney disorders, or a history of urinary tract infections are especially susceptible to the destructive action of fluoride on their bones and internal organs. So why are we using it?

Organized medicine endorsed fluoridation of public water supplies about 25 years ago but they did it hastily and without adequate research. Who really decided fluoride was good for us. Well consider this: in 1951 the Aluminum Company of America troubled with lawsuits by farmers who accused them of fluoride pollution realized they could no longer dump their waste pollution into the land and water surrounding their plant so they advertised their waste sodium fluoride in chemical trade journals with a hand holding a glass of water inscribed, "Fluoride your water with confidence. Use high purity Alcoa Sodium Fluoride."

Today the fertilizer companies find it profitable to convert their fluoride waste into hydrofluosilicic acid and sell it as a fluoridating agent. They have to ship it in neoprene-lined tank trucks to avoid calamitous corrosion. So if industry can't dump fluoride in our water and on our land then why not dump it directly into us and make us pay for it to boot.

Some well-known people who have warned us against the use of excess fluoride are French oceanographer, Jacques Cousteau, consumer rights advocate Ralph Nader, cancer researcher, Dr. Dean

Burk, former head of the National Cancer Institutes cytochemitry section, and Dr. John Yiamouyiannis, science editor of the National Health Federation. Dr. Burk was quoted as saying, "One American drops dead every 20 minutes because of artificial fluoridation."

AVOID FLUORIDATED WATER

Do not confuse Sodium Fluoride with any cell salts. Fluoridated water contains Sodium Fluoride which is in fact the principle ingredient in rat poison. The unanswered question is: "Why is Sodium Fluoride in our city water any safer than it is in rat poison? Why is it there at all since it is Calcium Fluoride, not Sodium Fluoride that is beneficial to good teeth. It is interesting to note that Stalin used it for his prison camps because it causes mental retardation and docileness. It makes people dumb.

I do not believe Sodium Fluoridated water is good for the general public.

How do we get rid of the fluoride in our water when it is already there? Well we can't boil it out but we can buy water filter devices that filter it out or bottled water. But with so many bottled waters on the market it is wise to read the labels of whatever you are buying. In my own home I drink a balance of distilled water and filtered tap water. My filter removes chlorine, fluoride and synthetic compounds such as asbestos and pesticides. Your drinking water should be neutral, that is pH 7.0 or slightly alkaline meaning higher than 7.0 up to 8.0. Distilled water should be steam distilled and not reverse osmosis or ion-exchanged. The reverse osmosis process may pick up lead, copper, rust or other debris depending on how old or clean the tubing is. Steam distilled water is the purest form available today.

In my research on water I found some more interesting facts about chlorine and flouridated water. Chlorinated water destroys Vitamin E and the good intestinal bacteria in the body. Fluoride inactivates certain enzymes and interferes with digestion. Anything that interferes with digestion or takes vitamins out of our body is going to age us faster than our normal rate. I try to drink distilled water whenever possible because I feel I get enough of the essential minerals from my food and supplements. Also, all water except distilled contains Carbonate of Lime and this collects in the body causing or helping to cause kidney and gall stones. If you have ever seen the way lime collects in a tea kettle you will know exactly what I mean.

If you are interested in more information on this subject, the Cancer Control Society has a book available entitled, "Fluoridation Cancer Link."

What makes matters even worse with our current drinking water is that about 500 different chemicals are somehow getting into it along with what is generally referred to as "nothing to worry about conventional pollution" like human waste, organic materials from food processing, toxic residues from industry and suspended solids that the rain picks up on its way to earth. In the 500 chemicals are deadly toxins from fertilizers, herbicides, fungicides, detergents, and something we hear a lot about lately, the atomic energy radio active waters. Of course this ages our bodies faster than they would normally.

Many people are afraid to drink distilled water because they worry about losing the beneficial minerals found in regular water. But the minerals in regular water are really insignificant compared to those found in food. And there is no way to separate the good minerals like calcium, magnesium, iron and sodium from bad ones like lead and cadmium. Some of the lead in our bodies is picked up when water travels through lead pipes and some comes from auto exhaust, but this is something we don't need.

Another benefit of distilled water is that it carries away any harmful toxins that might be in the system. Drinking distilled water, especially after middle age, is helpful in delaying the aches and pains the body accumulates with unwanted mineral deposits. Most nutritionists advise drinking at least 6 glasses of water a day. I recommend drinking 8 glasses a day but this liquid intake can be in the form of teas or soups. Of course I recommend herb teas.

In the area of diet are certain food additives that cause internal body stress. Usually we think of stress as coming from outside the body but additives such as Monosodium Glutamate, Nitrites, Nitrates and Thyramine put the body through internal tension.

Monosodium Glutamate or MSG is a food additive that has been reported as causing headache, numbness and even chest pains. This is often called the "Chinese restaurant syndrome." If you like Chinese food and are allergic to MSG you can request the restaurant not to put MSG in your food. You have nothing to lose by asking except maybe a headache.

Nitrites and nitrates also cause headache in some people but they have recently been reported as possible cancer causing agents. Many processed meats contain these substances.

These dangerous additives cause more than transitory symptoms. Laboratory experiments showed brain damage, stunted skeletal development, sterility and obesity in mice injected with MSG. Experiments have shown that excessive nitrates accumulate in the stems and leaves of plants. Commercially grown vegetables frequently contain too much nitrate. Healthy people do excrete most nitrates out but they are toxins and do cause body stress. Nitrite can clump the blood hemoglobin and destroy its ability to carry oxygen from the lungs to the tissues. When our tissues die we age fast.

CHAPTER 10
Food Irradiation

In a book called "Food Irradiation, Who Wants It?" by Tony Webb, Tim Lang and Kathleen Tucker (Thorsons Publ.) it is reported that according to a study conducted by the National Institute of Nutrition at the Medical Research Center in Hyderbad, India, children fed freshly irradiated wheat developed polyploidy, a defect in the chromosomes of the blood cells. Polyploidy, frequently seen in cancerous tumor cells, is a significant health issue.

Also stated in this book is that food irradiation plants are powered by Cobalt 60 and Cesium 137. As part of their waste management program, the Department of Energy is preparing to finance, with $10 million, six irradiation demonstration plants, in the hopes that they can find some commercial value for their large supplies of nuclear waste. Disposal of radioactive Cesium 137 currently presents a considerable problem because of the quantities produced and the time it takes to decay.Cesium is a byproduct of nuclear reactor technology and has a 30 year life cycle. The authors of this book ask, "Could it be that the whole program to promote food irradiation is little more than a thinly disguised attempt to find a commercial use for radioactive waste?"

I ask the same thing about the push to fluoridate our water.

Opponents of food irradiation cite as problems the loss of vitamin potency, unpleasant odors, and flavors, and most importantly, changes in the molecular structure of treated foods. Irradiation kills bacteria and gives a longer shelf life but it doesn't remove toxins made by those bacteria. In studies conducted in 1976 and 78, observers noted the increased production of aflatoxins in foods following irradiation.Aflatoxins are powerful agents known for causing liver cancer.

The Food and Drug Administration has approved irradiation for pork, fruits, spices, and vegetables and is considering extending this to fish and poultry. The FDA permits food irradiation in doses as high as 100,000 rads. In comparison, a standard chest X-Ray consists of a fraction of one rad. Still the AMA, the USDA and the DOE defend food irradiation and in fact are assisting in the funding of new irradiation plants in California, Florida, Hawaii, Iowa, Oklahoma and Washington.

For the manufacturers and purveyors of food, the main aim is to extend the time that food can remain in storage, in transport and in stores before the customer buys it. Thus food manufacturers, especially those engaged in international trade, have the most to gain. The list comprising the Coalition For Food Irradiation includes some of the world's leading food manufacturers; Beatrice Companies, Inc., Del Monte Corp., General Foods, Gerber Products Co., Heinz USA, Hershey Foods Corp., Oscar Mayer Foods Corp., and Welch Foods Inc.

HAIR DYES

There have been reports that hair dyes can cause cancer but smoking or driving a car is far riskier than dyeing your hair. However, the National Cancer Institute has labeled seven coal-tar dyes, mostly used in the darker hair colorings as being potentially carcinogenic. Many hair dyes contain one or a combination of these dyes. A consumer group called The Environmental Defense Fund offers a list of all dyes that have suspected chemicals. The Environmental Defense Fund last known address was 1525 18th St. N.W., Washington, D.C. 20036. Although normally, most women do not have to worry about this as very few women have the kind of skin that seems capable of absorbing any significant amount of the dye.

In skin tests done on rats and mice at the Eppley Institute for Cancer at the University of Nebraska there has been no finding of cancer. At the National Cancer Institute laboratories, the rats that did get cancer had been given large daily doses of hair dyes in their food. But how many of us eat hair dyes?

Some health food stores carry hair dye products. Anyone who might be worried about hair dyes should check these out.

CHAPTER 11
Internal Body Cleansing

Every year, according to the National Cancer Institute 100,000 people die from colon cancer. Colon cancer is the second leading malignancy in the United States with 102,000 new cases every year. Rather frightening statistics, but how can a person tell when they have a problem in this area? Very often the face starts to wrinkle excessively and this means there is degenerative trouble beginning inside the body. To use an analogy it is like your insides are the "Portrait of Dorian Gray." And if you don't know what that means it is simply a person who looks better on the outside than on the inside.

This is a direct result of the type of food we put into our bodies and the amount of stress we are subjected to daily. Perhaps we can't do too much about the stress but we certainly can stop putting highly processed, refined, sugared and salted so called food into our system because this will eventually clog up our colons the same way sludge accumulates in a car's engine.

When it really gets bad, we develop toxemia, diverticulitis, spastic colon, constipation, dropped transverse of the large intestine and that very familiar problem, hemorrhoids. This is just naming a few of the possible aggravations.

So be aware of these signs: thin, inelastic, dry skin; pigmentations of yellow, brown, black, blue or general muddy complexion; problems with sores, boils, herpes, eczema, dermatitis, lupus erythmarosus, acne rosacrea, psoriasis and jaudice. Any constant problem with the skin is a sign of internal body problems. Lupus erythemarosus will show up as red scaly patches on the skin. Degenerations of muscles of any part of the body, includes not only the facial muscles and below, but the internal heart and joint muscles as well.

The colon is a natural breeding ground for bacteria, and there are two types of bacteria; the healthy scavenger type known as bacilli coli and the pathogenic or disease-producing kind. In a clean colon the healthy bacteria will control the pathogenic kind.

The very purpose of the colon is to collect all fermative and putrefactive toxic waste from every part of the body and by the peristaltic wave of the muscles of the colon remove all solid and semi-solid waste from the body. In simple words the colon is the sewage system of the body. The health of the colon affects the health of the body. The use of laxatives and cathartics are not only habit forming but destructive to the membranes of the intestine. They disturb the normal rhythm of the excretory organs, which can lead to a one way street . . . a colostomy.

As stated, bowel cancer ranks No. 2 among cancer deaths. One of the best procedures for maintaining a friendly healthy flora is acidophilus. Besides aiding in the preparation of waste material for excretion from the body, the friendly germs also produce vitamin B12 for the body's use. The intestinal environment induced by lactobacillus also inhibits parasites and generates hydrogen peroxide, which help to "activate" intestinal germs and harmful bacteria."

Antibiotics can destroy the colonies of acidophilus so it is wise for anyone using them to take supplemental acidophilus. As stated previously, acidophilus is safe to take.

KYO-DOPHILUS

There's a war going on in our bodies as you read this book. It's the same old story — the good guys versus the bad guys. It's taking place in your intestines . . . between the friendly bacteria that fight disease and putrefaction and the unfriendly bacteria that produce toxins.

Lactic acid and acetic acid feed the friendly bacteria and give them the vitality and strength to detoxify our bodies. They are our security agents — our lifesavers.

Lactic acid is necessary for the vitality and growth of new cells — the very seeds of life. Each little cell in the body is constantly engaged in the life-renewal process of taking in food and oxygen and throwing off waste products. This process depends on the presence of certain lactic acid ferments.

Unfortunately, antibiotics and stress play havoc with the balance of bacteria in our bodies. The antibiotics not only kill the bad guys but devastate the good guys too — and that's where many of our health problems begin.

One of the best products to take to restore our friendly bacteria is Kyo-Dophilus. Kyo-Dophilus manufactures B vitamins, including B6 which helps keep the cholesterol-count down. Kyo-Dophilus is three superior strains of bacteria. L. Acidophilus, B. Bifidus, and S. faecalis. Kyo-Dophilus is heat-stable (no refrigeration is needed) and implants quickly throughout the entire digestive tract. Kyo-Dophilus produces both lactic and acetic acids and is presently used in over 30,000 hospitals and clinics.

Kyo-Dophilus is distributed in health food stores and is recommended by many doctors for their Candida patients. Kyo-Dophilus helps keep our intestinal garden flourishing and does wonders in normalizing our internal plumbing (regularity).

Kyo-Dophilus inhibits the growth of unfriendly bacteria and promotes a healthy digestive tract. Because of the variety of foods we eat, our digestive tract contains more than 100 different species of micro-organisms numbering in the billions.

Kyo-Dophilus works together to promote the body's defense system, reduce waste in the intestinal tract, and form acids that prevent the spread of harmful micro-organisms. Kyo-Dophilus is completely safe and so superior that young children in Japan are given it for the promotion of digestive health.

Kyo-Dophilus must be taken after meals — it survives the stomach acids and retains its beneficial properties when tested at 120° F. for 6 months. No other product tested could come close to surviving under these conditions. Most products at room temperature lost 99 percent of their viability in less than 14 days.

Many problems arising with arthritis, bursitis and lumbago can be directly traced to poisons in the colon. Constant headaches and other body pains are also symptoms.

The eyes have often been referred to as the mirror of the soul but they can also mirror the body's insiders as well. Degenerative changes in the eye, inflammation of the lens and/or optic nerve, hardening of the lens, sclerotitis, iritis, cataract, recurrent hemorrhage in the retina and dull heavy feelings in the eyes are also some of the ways the body tries to tell you it needs a good housecleaning.

Very often we don't realize how bad the inside looks because we manage to function fairly well; maybe we need a little help from a laxative, aspirin, sedative or pain pill once in a while but isn't that pretty normal? The answer is No, that is not normal. The best way to get rid of many of the bodies problems is to start with a good body cleansing from the inside out. Either oxygen and water colonics or the good old-fashioned enema, or a combination of both.

Unfortunately, there are not too many places where one can find a competent oxygen and water colonic clinic. The usual way to get this type of treatment is through a chiropractic clinic.

The basic principle behind the oxygen and water colonic is to clean the colon of debris that might be causing harmful bacteria to infiltrate into the entire system. The water cleans out the waste material and the oxygen heals sores that may have been caused by irritation in the colon. The colon is also known as the large intestine. Some people frown on this because they claim the good bacteria is cleaned out with the bad but as I have explained it is very easy to replace the good bacteria with the help of kyodophilus, yogurt, whey, buttermilk or raw natural kefir plus various supplements.

If one decides to go through a series of these colonics there is usually an entire program to follow during the time involved. It would include a good food diet and certain exercises that would stimulate the colon muscles to work more effectively.

However, if an oxygen and water colonic is not available then you can do almost as good a job with home style herbal or coffee enemas. I believe the best ones to get started with are either the garlic or the coffee enema. Both cause a peristalsis contraction and relaxation of the colon by which the contents are forced through the system and eliminated.

The procedure is simple. With coffee, perk or drip regular, let it cool and use 2 quarts of lukewarm coffee water.

GARLIC ENEMA

Use Kyolic liquid garlic. Two tablespoons of liquid garlic to 2 quarts of warm water. This will cause oxygen to accumulate in the colon and you may have some gas discomfort for an hour. But it's a good colon cleanser and worth the discomfort once in a while. You'll have to be judge of how often.

Usually it takes about 10 to 12 enemas, one a day to do a proper job. The last three days the enema solution should be changed to a more healing combination like chlorophyll, chamomile or comfrey tea or a combination of all three. Chlorophyll liquid is available in a health food store.

During this time it is best to refrain from eating heavily or from eating flesh or processed foods. Try to maintain a fairly liquid diet with both fruit and vegetable juices plus different vegetable soups. This isn't as difficult as it may sound, in fact it's a great time to lose excess poundage or bloat.

One of the exercises to stimulate the body to eliminate toxins is to roll the feet over a wooden rolling pin or better yet there is a Weihs-Roller available that massages thoroughly. It is square shaped with six rows of wooden rollers. It can not only be used for feet but for abdomen, back and leg also. You can roll your feet over it while sitting on the toilet or you can set the roller on the floor and roll your back over it.

Another good back massager is a medium sized rubber ball from any toy store or drug store. Roll your backbone up and down while lying on the ball and you will find it helpful in aligning the bones if they are only stiff from bad posture. This little trick has saved me from many backaches and doctor bills.

Another method that helps to straighten the backbone is hanging from a door. Throw a towel over the door top so your hands don't get dents.

SKIN BRUSHING

Brushing the skin with a natural bristle body

brush or complexion brush for the face brings blood to the skin surface and helps the circulation to bring oxygen to the cells. This also helps eliminate toxins from the skin.

During a period of cleansing it is important to eat garlic and onions and the easiest way to do this is to include them in your soups. During the cleansing period it is important to include kyodophilus at least twice a day, about two tablespoons, plus a tablespoon of chlorophyll liquid three times a day and 8 glasses of distilled water throughout the day.

Sometimes I grow my own chlorophyll by planting wheat grass in a window box in my backyard. Within a week the grass is about 4 inches high and I cut some off, put it in a serrated bowl and grind it with a wooden grinder until it's a deep green color. Then I drink it and sometimes I chew a small amount of grass and swallow it. It's not the same type of grass that grows on your lawn. Wheat grass will grow up again 3 or 4 times before it has to be dumped and new seeds planted. Chlorophyll brings oxygen to the body cells.

Aloe Vera Gel is also a fine body cleanser. It contains Vitamin C, Amino Acids and enzymes that help rejuvenate aged tissue and promote healthy skin. Two tablespoons a day are recommended for cleansing. Aloe also soothes the pain of ulcers.

It's best not to do strenuous exercise during your cleansing period, but walking is fine or swimming if weather permits.

Some people get a euphoric feeling during a cleansing period. It's a natural high and it starts them off in the right direction toward healthier lives.

However, during this time span you may feel slightly weak or even nauseous for the first few days. That may be because the body is cleansing itself of toxins so fast that they're being thrown back into the system before it can eliminate them. This is nothing to worry about. One man I know could never give up smoking until he went through this cleansing period then he couldn't even stand the smell of someone else's smoke.

When coming off a cleansing regimen it is very important to eat the right foods. Start with raw fruits and vegetables the first couple of days then switch to vege-burgers instead of hamburgers. Then if you return to flesh foods begin with fish or chicken as they are more easily digested than red meats.

People who are accustomed to eating lots of meat are often concerned about getting enough protein. As I have explained there are plenty of products with sufficient protein. Just eat whole grains, nuts, seeds, brown rice, beans and dairy products. If you combine nuts, seeds and legumes you'll get an excellent balance of amino acids. This is the principle of combining and complimenting proteins for optimum utilization.

One last word on colonics and enemas. I want to make it clear that not everybody needs them. If one has been health conscious most of their life and refrained from eating too much meat, refined sugars and starches, and processed foods that have either been injected with chemicals or had all the necessary vitamins and minerals crushed out then there would be no need for a colonic and enema program.

However, if you don't want to rely on your physically visible signs then have a barium x-ray taken of your large intestine. This type of service is also found through a chiropractic clinic. But when it comes to x-rays, I do not believe in having any more than are absolutely necessary. If the technician wants you to have more than one just refuse and remind them that x-rays are accumulative. One x-ray will usually tell you exactly what kind of shape you are really in.

Remember certain foods will help correct constipation. Sufficient residue and roughage are in fresh fruits, vegetables, bran, fresh ground flax seeds, psyllium seed or powder, raw pumpkin seeds, kelp, alfalfa and cayenne pepper assure exercise for the intestinal tract. This helps to stimulate food transit time and facilitate cleansing of the bowel lining, protecting against toxemia and diseases that begin in the colon.

And on the subject of food I interviewed the owner of a health food restaurant, an ambassador of good will and good health and the owner of a health food store.

HEALTH FOOD RESTAURANTS

Nowadays health food restaurants are fairly common but 20 years ago they were extremely rare. A pioneer in nutritionally conscious restaurants is a retired dentist named Dr. Robert I. Franks. His Old World restaurants in Los Angeles, California are a favorite with the health aware public. Dr. Franks had a flourishing dental practice for over 40 years. When I interviewed him for this book one of the first things he said was, "A person today must be knowledgeable about their health because our current so called civilization doesn't suit us as human beings and the result is bad health physically and mentally.

If you don't have the right nutrients in your body, your brain won't function and that's why we have so many street people today. If the government was really interesed in its people they would clean up the environment, stop spraying pesticides, stop dumping pollutants everywhere and make our soil rich enough to give us back the foods that are filled with vitamins and minerals.

I have to seek out organic farmers and make a real effort to find food that isn't sprayed with chemicals and grown in poor soil.

Really if our government would make an effort to clean up our environment they would save billions that they spend on social and drug problems. What could stop a lot of our drug problems is not legislation but education and good nutriton. Teach the kids how wonderful their bodies are, show them how they can look and feel their best and show them the bad things that can destroy their bodies and their brains."

When I asked him how he felt about the new "No Smoking" ordinance in Beverly Hills he replied, "I think they should have a "No Smoking" rule everywhere. There are up to 6,000 chemicals in cigarette smoke to say nothing about the fact that putting smoke in your lungs is detrimental to your well-being. No one who really cares about themselves should smoke. Really what is more important, money or health? Go ask a millionaire who is dying of lung cancer the answer to that question. If he's still in his right mind he'd say he'd give up all his money to have his health back."

Dr. Franks went on to explain, "I became a dentist because my own teeth were bad. My mother never breast fed me and I knew nothing about nutrition until I was 25 years old. You know it is very important to be breast fed, not only does it help your immune system and nourish your body but it also helps to give you a good jaw and proper teeth development. It wasn't until my senior year in dental college that a professor told me there was a relationship between teeth decay, bone structure breaking down and diabetes from the over-consumption of refined carbohydrates.

"About 20 years ago a doctor told me to expect prostate problems in my sixties and possible prostate cancer in my eighties. Well I just wouldn't accept that. I'm 85 now and I've never had a prostate problem. Also have all my teeth but if I hadn't become knowledgeable about nutrition I probably would have been dead in my late 40's because I sure didn't have a good beginning."

I said, "You believe you saved yourself?"

He nodded, "Yes, and I believe everybody has to save themselves. We must keep our immune systems strong. There will always be germs and viruses in the air but if we have a strong immune system they won't harm us."

"If our government encouraged good health and educated its people towards that goal they could save billions on health care and we wouldn't have to constantly build bigger hospitals."

So what's the average day like for this 85 year old youngster? Well, besides running his restaurants, he swims every morning, then has a half a lemon with 2 tablespoons of black strap molasses or pure maple syrup, in a glass of water, then a tablespoon of Cod Liver Oil and a couple of oranges which he peels and eats the whole pieces, then a protein drink with 2 tablespoons of oat bran and a raw egg. He has no fear of eggs and may have up to 3 a day. He said, "Eggs have all the amino acids plus lecithin which is a natural emulsifier of cholesterol. Also pectin lowers cholesterol. Apples have pectin. Try to eat eggs from chickens that run around the ground and are not cooped up under artificial lights. Fertile eggs are good and the best way to eat them is soft boiled, poached or raw. And don't worry about cholesterol. If you don't have enough cholesterol your body will manufacture its own."

He eats a lot of green salads and has a diet which consists of whole grains, seeds, nuts, fruits and fish from the north Atlantic because the rest of the oceans are polluted. He eats a minimum of meats, and when he eats desserts they are made from honey, molasses, turbinado sugar and fruits. But if he has to make a choice between sugar and a sugar substitute he will take the sugar because the body can not metabolize chemicals. Anything the body can't metabolize (digest) causes it harm.

There is a big difference between regular white sugar and honey. Honey has trace minerals and helps the body use calcium more efficiently, it improves the red blood cell count and is rich in aspartic acid, essential for rejuvenation.

Dr. Franks' philosophy for a long and healthy life. "Try to stay so healthy that you never have to see a doctor or a hospital unless you have an accident.

Because most of the drugs doctors prescribe do more harm to the body than good and they break down the immune system. Be sure to read a lot and never stop educating yourself and being interested in life."

GYPSY BOOTS

"Gypsy Boots" has become a legend in his own time!

At 77 years of age, Southern California's most eccentric health nut is still going strong. Running all over town, spouting corny poems, giving away organic fruit, throwing footballs with 50-yard bullet passes, and forever flirting with the ladies. Gypsy is an inspiration to those of us who, while trying to embrace a healthy lifestyle, sometimes wonder if the extra efforts will pay off in later years.

Gypsy became a nationally known character as a regular on the Steve Allen Show in the 1960's, never failing to throw the studio into an uproar with his outrageous antics. He has written two books, *"Bare Feet and Good Things To Eat"* and *"How To Stay Young At Any Age"* (packed with hilarious stories, healthy recipes, and pictures of himself with celebrities and famous athletes) which, together, have sold over 200,000 copies.

Gypsy exercises every day, stretching, doing squats, lifting rocks, playing tennis with superstars, and running barefoot through Ferndale Park. At age 77, he has the physique of a college athlete. He eats 90% raw foods. The only cooked foods he eats are steamed vegetables. *"I eat a lot of corn,"* he said, *"maybe that's why I'm so corny."* Plus lots of greens and green juices. He doesn't eat any dairy products, except for some occasional goat milk with Medjool dates. He discovered years ago that garlic was an excellent detoxifier, and began eating raw cloves of garlic regularly. That smelly habit cost him five girlfriends and a job with the Spike Jones Band. Since then he's discovered Kyolic, an odorless garlic extract from Japan, he has become an enthusiastic fan, and believes that Kyolic helped him cure his arthritis. Kyolic is marketed through Wakunaga of America Co., Ltd., 23501 Madero, Mission Viejo, California 92691.

Gypsy Boots" is a free spirit with a healthy sense of humor. He doesn't get older — just better even at the age of 77. Gypsy still runs like a deer, jumps like a kangaroo and swings from trees like a gorilla.

The National Athletic Health Institute gave Gypsy a physical fitness evaluation and here is a summary of their results.

"The functional capacity of your heart is extraordinary. Your oxygen consumption, which is considered to be the most precise index of total fitness by a majority of researchers in the field of exercise physiology — is above the minimum level of 50ml/kg/min which we recommend for most professional athletes. Your level of fitness both in respect to endurance and strength are remarkable in consideration of your age."

I've known Gypsy Boots for over 25 years and I marvel at his overflowing vitality. He is truly an ambassador of good health and natural living.

MRS. GOOCH'S NATURAL FOOD MARKET

The first Mrs. Gooch's Natural Food Market opened in 1977 in Southern California. By 1987 they were recognized as the leading natural foods retail supermarkets in the country. How did this come to happen in such a short period of time? Simple, if you give the people what they want they'll beat a path to your door.

Mrs. Gooch's Natural Foods Markets are the result of a near death experience of one of its owners, Sandy Gooch. In 1974, Sandy was a wife, mother, school teacher and homemaker and was in good physical health except for an allergy to peanut products. She woke up one day with sniffles and her doctor prescribed tetracyline, a commonly used antibiotic. But a few days later she thought she was dying with severe chest pains and her head spinning she felt like she was having a heart attack. She was rushed to an emergency hospital but the doctors could find nothing wrong. Eventually her symptoms subsided but two weeks later she had an eye infection and was given tetracyline again. Within minutes her body was under siege again and the struggle lasted for three days. Frightened by this she went to the Scripps Clinic and Research Foundation in La Jolla where she underwent treatment for ten days. On the fifth day, while doctors were observing her symptoms, another attack occurred but they managed to bring it under control with a shot of Benadryl. Mrs. Gooch feels their timely presence saved her life.

But when she left the hospital she was panic stricken that the attacks might happen again so she consulted with her father, a research biologist and he began his own investigation. She recalled that the last thing she had swallowed prior to her seizure was a popular diet soft drink. Her father contacted the company to find out more about the ingredients in that drink. It contained bromelated vegetable oil or bromelated acetate, as this ingredient is scientifically defined, and that is an instant antihistamine reducer. It inhibits the body's natural antihistamine defenses which are needed to fight infections and allergies. Yet it is considered by the FDA to be fit for human consumption. At the time of her attack her body was in a weakened condition from the tetracyline. That drug had lodged in her liver and kidneys and continued to seep out through her system and the diet soda had further depleted her body's supply of antihistamines. The combination nearly cost her life as the enzymes working towards the production of her antihistamines were paralyzed by the ingestion of the soft drink.

Through this negative experience she found that she was one of many people who suffer from the effects of processed foods. She began asking questions, reading labels and lots of literature about additives and ingredients in food. She began her search for pure, additive-free foods, an alternative to the prepacked convenience fare sold in most conventional supermarkets. When she saw how difficult it was to find good pure foods she began to explore the idea of creating a store that would stock only natural foods that were healthy and free from harmful ingredients.

It seemed a pipe dream for she had been a school teacher for 17 years and then a housewife and her knowledge of the business world was very limited. She approached a natural food store manager named Dan Volland who had management experience and source buying experience and they became partners. The rest is history.

Today Mrs. Gooch is again in the forefront of the health industry. This time in the battle against food irradiation. In December 1985, the Department of Health and Human Services approved a proposal to allow irradiation of fresh fruits and vegetables in order to control insects, inhibit spoilage and extend shelf life. Up until now irradiation treatment has been permitted in the U.S. only on a limited number of food products.

Most people in the health industry who are knowledgeable on the subject do not believe food irradiation is healthy for humans.

Also in the fight against food irradiation is the National Food Assn. They are trying to educate the public on the possible injurious consequences to their health. People who care about their food supply should make their preferences known to food merchants and store managers. As stated Americans have unknowingly been eating irradiated foods processed at relatively low radiation levels for the past three years in the form of herbs, spices, pork, wheat, some potatoes and some prepared foods like pizza and cookies. Fortunately there are some foods that do not irradiate well like leafy greens they tend to lose their green color, grapes become soft and bananas develop brown spots.

But it's like Mrs. Gooch says, "Buyer beware. Read labels, ask questions and for your health's sake fight back by not buying products that are not good for you. That's why we work with a variety of scientists and medical doctors in developing our own label products so that we can be sure the ingredients are pure and healthful. We get our meats from an organic rancher in Colorado named Mel Coleman.

Our fish is fresh and we don't dip it in any preservatives like Sodium Benzoate."

Also involved in the health business, Mrs. Gooch's husband Harry Lederman told me that when they travel they take along a little "Survival Kit" that includes: Vitamin C, Beta Carotene, A to B Calm which is a Calcium and Magnesium supplement, Liquid Kyolic Garlic and capsules, Herbal C Emergen-C by Alacer (Sylvester Stallone credits this for helping him get through the rigors of movie making) Charcoal Tablets, Aloe Vera, Sun Chlorella, Ginseng, Cyclone Cider and Honey LoQuats for sore throat, Primrose Oil, Solgars Multiple Vitamin, Thompsons Multiple for children and Waleeda mouthwash. Harry says this whole medical kit can be carried in a shoulder flight bag.

CHAPTER 12
X-Rays

On January 9, 1987 in the Los Angeles Times newspaper an article appeared about Chemotherapy by Martin Shapiro, an internist and associate professor of medicine at UCLA. There were two paragraphs that I found quite interesting. Here's what he said: "Chemotherapy is a serious undertaking. It often causes hair loss, severe nausea, vomiting, bone-marrow suppression with associated hemorrhaging, infections and death. The only reason for chemotherapy should be to cure cancer, prolong life or relieve symptoms. For some cancers, such as leukemia, lymphomas, breast and testicular cancer, chemotherapy accomplishes one or more of these objectives."

"Unfortunately, for four of the most common kinds of cancer, colon and rectum, pancreas, stomach and most kinds of lung cancer, there is no convincing evidence that chemotherapy offers any benefit whatsoever. Yet many people with these types of cancers are being treated with chemotherapy, and are not aware that they are subjecting themselves to considerable risks, discomfort and expense for no perceptible benefit. (It should be noted that a small proportion of these cancers can be cured by surgical removal of the tumor, and patients may obtain some relief of symptoms with radiation therapy.)"

Many times a patient is not informed about the effectiveness of a certain treatment and if the information is not forthcoming from the doctor then it is up to the patient to seek it out.

Speaking about cancer therapy treatments the late Dr. Max Gerson said, "My own experiences show that the majority of patients who had 40 to 80 deep x-ray treatments and, in addition, 16 to 40 cobalt treatments could not recover at all."

Every time I have to have an x-ray I increase my dosage of Ester-C before and after the X-ray. Generally I will take about 5000 mg. that day spacing them out at 1000 mg. each hour the first hour or two before exposure and 1000 mg. each hour after the exposure. A lot of research has gone into showing us the protective benefits of Vitamin C from Linus Pauling to Irwin Stone, D.SC., a biochemist and author of "The Healing Factor: Vitamin C Against Disease" Grosset and Dunlap, 1972. In fact, it was Dr. Stone who first suggested to Linus Pauling that he take Vitamin C as it helps to shield the body against the lethal poisons of cigarette smoke. That led Pauling into his studies of Vitamin C as a simple and effective means of preventing the common cold.

Now there seems to be a lot of hype to get women over 35 to have annual mammograms. I do not believe in annual mammograms as a preventive against cancer. Just as I did not believe taking an annual chest x-ray was a good idea. Unless you suspect that you have something wrong or unless you feel a lump in your breast that needs to be checked then I say annual x-rays are needless radiation accumulation. We get enough fallout radiation from nuclear tests, nuclear power plant disasters, from our own government and foreign governments and from so-called harmless low level radiation from high voltage lines, smoke detectors, TV and radio transmitters, diathermy machines, burglar alarms, garage door openers and microwave ovens and now food irradiation!

For 11½ years the American government exploded 84 Atomic bombs above ground in Nevada until an international agreement banned such tests. People in the surrounding Nevada and Utah area reported an increase of cancer and it is interesting to note that Hollywood was making a film in Nevada at that time and several people working on the film died of cancer including the stars Susan Hayward and John Wayne. We are still exploding A-bombs underground.

When people march and protest against this our government arrests them. It sure makes me wonder who's in charge and if they don't have any brains then their common sense should tell them exploding atomic bombs is wrong.

With all the cancer work and cancer research that has been done in the last 20 years there has been no appreciable decrease in cancer. In fact, the U.S. Cancer Research Council in Wash., D.C. reports that in 1982, one out of five died of cancer, in 1986 one out of three and they predict that by 1990 one out of two will die of cancer. Of the estimated 870,000 people who will get cancer this year, 50% will die, that's 435,000 people, most of whom were probably getting the latest in medical treatment for cancer.

X-RAYS

While we are on the subject of x-rays I'd like to say a little about the safety limit of medical and dental x-rays. In view of the increasing sources of radiation in this nuclear age we now live in it is wise to be cautious about how much radiation we get individually.

In a book entitled "A Cancer Therapy" by the late Max Gerson, M.D. he also stated that it is wise for everyone to keep a personal record of x-rays taken. As a general population safety limit exposure to radiation should be held down to 10 roentgens for the first 30 years of a person's life. A roentgen is a unit for measuring the harmful gamma ray from medical and dental x-ray equipment, nuclear weapons explosions and from natural causes like cosmic rays and natural radium. Obstetricians who take x-rays of pregnant women are exposing the baby to 3 or 4 roentgens. Too much radiation causes mutation or harmful changes in the genes or germ cells of the reproductive organs. Damage manifests itself in shortening the life span, reducing the ability to produce children and sometimes, not often, produces deformed children. Even if the mutation is in one gene, that mutation will go on through every generation until the line that bears it becomes extinct. Mutant genes can only disappear when the inheritance line in which they are carried dies out. In cases of severe and obvious damage this may happen in the first generation, in other cases it may require hundreds of generations. For the general population, a little radiation to a lot of people is as harmful as a lot of radiation to a few, since the total number of mutant genes can be the same in both cases.

Every time we get a medical or dental x-ray a certain amount of radiation is sustained by our sex organs. There currently exists no way of measuring how much and it is generally believed that if that area is shielded the exposure is less. A dental x-ray delivers about 0.005 roentgens to the gonads. A general fluoroscopic examination 2 or 3 or more roentgens.

Again common sense tells us there is something drastically wrong with all of this. We can be sure of one thing, the latest medical treatments bring in billions to the drug companies, the hospitals and the medical profession.

The best prevention against cancer is a healthy diet, a moderate amount of exercise, good mental outlook (that means turning the negative to positive, keeping a sense of humor) and keeping our stress level down to a quiet roar . . . which is all most of us can do in todays world.

CHAPTER 13

Safe Sex

Thank God for Dr. Ruth! Long may she reign over the constantly confused couples. I remember in college hearing a young man wail, "I'm dying to get laid." Today that could be the literal truth. Casual sex with a partner you don't know well is really playing Russian Roulette.

First America was in a Victorian era with a very strict sexual code of conduct and basically that continued right through the 1950's but then came the pill and society decided it was time to break the traditional bonds of matrimony and we went into the swinging 60's with so-called "free love" and hog wild promiscuity. That lasted right through the 70's and even Herpes didn't stop it, maybe slowed it down a little bit but swinging and promiscuity was still going strong in the 80's when suddenly along came a new virus called AIDS which brought promiscuity and swinging to a screeching halt.

Now everyday we are bombarded with new information and frightening statistics about AIDS. However, so many people still have misinformation about AIDS that instead of those initials standing for Acquired Immune Deficiency Syndrome they seem to stand for Acquired Idiot Dingbat Syndrome. But for anyone interested in avoiding AIDS here is the latest information on how to reduce your chances of getting it.

AVOID CASUAL SEX

Discrimination is desirable in the 1990's. Avoid casual sex. Know your partner well. If engaged in oral sex, don't swallow semen. Don't rim. Tongue and mouth contact with the anus results in a high intake of viruses, bacteria and parasites which can cause infection and lower immunity to all kinds of disease.

Don't insert objects: i.e. dildoes, fists, into the rectum, that can tear the delicate lining and lead to infection and injury. Anal intercourse is not advised, but if having it use a condom. Any direct contact with feces increases exposure to many diseases. Don't drink urine, it also contains viruses.

SPERM MAY CAUSE CANCER

During intercourse viruses from sperm can enter the blood stream. Studies have shown that sperm may be a cause of cancer. Ellen Borenfreud, a biochemist at the Memorial Sloan-Kettering Cancer Center, says that spermatozoa may be linked to cancer of the prostate in men and cervical cancer in women. The prostate is the second most frequent site of cancer in men, while the cervix is the fourth most frequent site of cancer in women. The biochemist reported that she introduced sperm from mice and rats into a culture dish containing somatic (body) cells. Some of the sperm penetrated the cells and induced changes that resulted in abnormal growths. The changes were similar to those that take place when cells are treated with carcinogens (cancer causing agents). Ms. Borenfreud speculates that sperm transports a virus or other cancer causing agents to the prostate or cervix. It is also possible that sperm itself may somehow upset the reproductive systems of individual cells, causing cancer.

It is interesting to note, that the cervical cancer rate is 2 to 4 times higher among Spanish speaking women. A University of Southern California physician, Dr. Duane E. Townsend believes that probable reason for this is that their culture encourages early marriages. Cancer authorities believe that intercourse at an early age increases the chances of acquiring the disease because the cervix is most sensitive to cancer in the middle and late teens. Dr. Townsend is Associate Professor of Obstetrics and Gynecology at the USC school of medicine.

I interviewed Dr. Howard R. Bierman, a specialist in hematology and oncology and he felt that an uncircumcised penis could be a carcinogenic agent because smegma bacillus, an accumulation of white mucuos type material, collects in the foreskin if not regularly washed and kept clean. Dr. Bierman said there is a sect in India called the Parsees that wash their genitals 4 times a day and very few cervical cancers are reported from them.

From the studies I have read, women who have

multiple male sex partners are also more prone to cervical cancer. Here, again, the condom would act as basic preventative medicine.

MORE OF AVOID LIST

Avoid Amyl Nitrite and Butyl Nitrite, popularly known as poppers; Cocaine, Marijuana and pills such as Qualudes, all of these can decrease your immunity to disease.

If you are not an alcoholic then alcohol can be taken in moderation. The old 2 drink minimum order should be a 2 drink maximum order.

AIDS SYMPTOMS

Some of the AIDS symptoms are swollen glands, weight loss, fever, fatique, diarrhea, bloody stool, sore throat, persistent cough, easy bruising or bleeding, rashes, blurred vision, and constant headaches. Many of us have had one or more of these symptoms at one time or another but if they do not go away after a normal amount of time, see your doctor.

THE IMMUNE SYSTEM

Our immune system is bombarded everyday by pollutants, irritants, radiation and chemicals we can not avoid in modern day society. That is why it is so important not to deliberately pollute or break down our immune system with things we could avoid, i.e. drugs, excess alcohol, pills, promiscuity and smoking.

Diseases such as Gonorrhea and Syphilis have pretty well been eliminated with antibiotics. However in early 1988 they were back in the news again. Health officials were reporting outbreaks at an alarming rate. But diseases such as Herpes, Chlamydia and Veneral Warts are a real pain in the butt. After Herpes became well known the joke was, "What's the difference between Herpes and love?" The answer, "Herpes lasts forever!"

Herpes are oral and/or genital cold sores, a virus that doesn't seem to go away. It will sleep in the body for awhile, but the minute one gets run down or stressed out Herpes can erupt again and then it is contagious. Some researchers have said it could be contagious during the dormant stage but usually that is not the case.

Again the reason that some people catch something and others do not is generally how strong is their immune system. The best way to build yourself up to resist disease so that you can live to laugh about life is with adequate rest, taking time for relaxation, eating a nutritionally sound diet, one that is right for you not necessarily the latest fad, and sometimes extra supplements of vitamins, minerals, herbs, cell salts and Bach flower remedies. There are always going to be "Sexy Food Lists" around with things like Garlic, Ginseng, oysters, parsley and seeds and these are foods that could enhance the sex drive but any good nutritional diet will enhance the sex drive.

Now what about the connection between fluoridation and AIDS? In a book entitled, "AIDS, Terror,Truth & Triumph," by Michael Culbert, D.Sc. published by the Bradford Foundation, Chula Vista, Calif. 1986, several studies were done on the connection between the statistics of AIDS and the cities with fluoridated water. Cities with fluoridation have a higher amount of AIDS cases. Two biochemists who believe there is a connection between

disease and fluoridation are Dr. John Yiamouyiannis, Ph.D. and Dr. Dean Burk, Ph.D. Dr. Burk is
recently retired from the National Cancer Institute.
Dr. Yiamouyiannis believes there is a direct connection between accelerated aging and fluoridation and
relates this in his book "The Aging Factor."

CHLAMYDIA

Chlamydia is the most prevalent sexually
transmitted disease and just like all the others the
more partners you have the more likely your chances
to contract it. The bacteria is similar to Gonorrhea in
that 80% of women and 50% of men show no symptoms. If you do have symptoms, it could be an in-
flamed cervix for women and/or painful urination
and discharge. Men could also have painful urination and discharge from the penis. Again your best
preventive is the condom and to know your sex
partner well.

VENEREAL WARTS

Venereal warts,or Condylomata acuminata,
haven't received much attention but they are another
common viral infection in both sexes. The virus is
called papilomaviruse which is a genital virus that
penetrates the skin of the anus and genitals and is
transmitted by sexual contact with someone who
carries the virus or who has veneral warts. The warts
are very contagious in their early stages but are less
so when they have been present for a long period of
time. However, more than half the people exposed
to a partners warts develop warts but the incubation
period of warts may stretch from 6 weeks to 8
months. These warts differ in structure from the
common type of skin warts that people get on their

fingers and other skin areas. Common skin warts do not usually affect the genital region.

In the female, veneral warts usually affect the skin of the vulva (vaginal lips) and the skin around the anus (opening to the rectum). They can also develop in the vagina and on the cervix. When they are present in the vagina and cervix, they can cause an abnormal Pap Smear. If they are the cause the Pap Smear will return to normal when the warts have been adequately treated. Venereal warts are not a form of cancer however they can break down the immune system and predispose an individual to cancer if they are vulnerable. In males, the warts can develop around or near the penis and the anus. The warts may itch or be irritated. Usually the first symptom a woman notices is a bump on the skin in the affected area. Unfortunately, some women may not have any symptoms. The warts frequently increase rapidly in size and number. For this reason, and to prevent infecting a sexual partner, they should be treated as soon as they are recognized.

Most cases of venereal warts can be treated easily with the application of Podophyllin, a solution which causes them to shrink over a number of days or weeks. In some cases, weekly applications may be necessary. Warts tend to recur, and if so, reapplication of the medication is necessary. This solution may cause some stinging and will irritate normal skin, so it is necessary to have a practitioner apply the medication each time.

Sadly, there is absolutely no effective way of preventing venereal warts. As with any venereal disease, using a condom during sexual activity is helpful. If exposure has taken place washing the vulva and/or penis with soap and water following sex may help prevent infection.

As for the cauliflower looking warts, there are over 25 known papillomaviruses but only 2 are thought to cause cervical cancer or to predispose one to the possibility of getting it.

USE YOUR HEAD

With all this frightening news about sexually transmitted disease you may be wondering if only YOU might be your best sexual partner!Or, perhaps, celibacy may be looking good even if you haven't joined a religious sect. Recently a men's magazine showed a picture of an erect penis with the caption underneath: "This head can't think so use yours!" I thought that ad very effective.

Well don't get too depressed, take heart but take precautions. Thinking first just may come back into style. Using condoms, chemical contraceptives, i.e. foams, cremes, jelly (Nonoxynol 9 is an ingredient found to be effective in killing germs including the AIDS virus) can not only prevent unwanted pregnancy but can prevent death as well.

KNOW YOUR OWN BODY

The only way to deal with today's sexual problems or for that matter with today's health problems in general is to literally become your own diagnostic doctor and a partner in your personal physicians care of you. Know your own body. Read current information. Be aware of what is happening in today's society and practice preventive medicine — that's the best kind of medicine available. If you do that, you can avoid that other contagious disease that seems to be an epidemic these days — it's called "AFRAIDS." Don't be afraid, just be aware.

BEST DRUG FOR SEX

For centuries man has been looking for a drug to enhance sexual performance never seeming to understand that the best drug for sex is LOVE. When you really love someone, everything about sex is enhanced. The type of hit and miss sex that a lot of men look for and some women too, is never as emotionally rewarding as really caring about somebody. Of course it is much more difficult to really care about someone than just to have sex with them. Just having sex has certainly caused a lot of problems . . . and many of them are walking around on two feet!

GOD'S PUNISHMENT

Interestingly, every time we have a sexually transmitted disease or some major plague we hear from the pulpits and various other pits that we are paying for our sins.

In the 14th century the Bubonic Plague killed 75 million people and it was popularly believed to be God's punishment for sin and as seems to happen more often than not it was blamed on the Jews! There were mass flagellations and mass purges of the Jews to appease the Lord. The actual cause of this plague was Asian fleas that traveled on the backs of rats via merchant ships bound for Europe.

Between 1832 and 1866 there was a cholera epidemic. Again this was hyped as a moral plague and a means of scourging humanity of sinners. Actually it was caused by bad sewage disposal, their sanitation department left much to be desired.

The influenza epidemic between 1917 and 1918 killed more than half a million Americans and was caused by air borne sneezes and coughs. Typhus also spread during that time caused by overcrowding in cities and unsanitary conditions contaminated water.

Smallpox caused by casual skin contact racked Europe for centuries and only since 1979 did the World Health Organization announce that it had been virtually wiped out.

All of this disease was believed by many to be God's way of scourging humanity of sinners. Well, if that was true, we would all be wiped out by now. I feel the worst plagues of all are not started by God but by ignorance and greed. Often disease is caused by the people who care more about profit than about people. The irony is that in their greed they will eliminate themselves, eventually, but usually they eliminate a lot of innocent people before that happens.

Even if some of us haven't learned by now that disease is NOT GOD'S PUNISHMENT for sin, we have learned that disease and plagues have been around for eons. But what seems to be changing is our ability to withstand the onslaught. Some say that is because the stress of our times is greater now than before but I don't believe that, each period of time has stress even going back to the cave man. I am sure that cave men and women were under a lot of stress trying to do the 4 minute mile running away from Dinosaurs.

So that brings us back to GREED which is often called PROGRESS. Progress has brought pollution. We like progress but we seem to hate cleaning up after ourselves. I see that at home all the time. I get more volunteers to help with the dinner than to help cleanup after. Still it always amazes me the way so many people trash their own environment, their own home. If only they would stop to realize that this environment, this planet, this earth is really their home and there is only one earth, one home, and all of us should be involved in keeping home clean.

I seem to spend a lot of time cleaning, not only my own immediate home but wherever I go, parks, beaches, walkways. Sometimes I wonder if I'm the only one who cares. The people in charge of chemical dumping don't seem to care, the ones who told us Nuclear Power plants would always be safe don't seem to care, the ones making engines and sprays that pollute the atmosphere and deteriorate our ozone don't seem to care, the people who throw their personal garbage anywhere don't seem to care and the one's that grafitti walls and destroy other people's property don't seem to care. As a kid in the 50's I remember a saying, "Fools names like fools faces are often seen in public places." Whenever I see someones name defacing a wall I think of that saying.

I suppose if you are not one of those in power you get frustrated and want to make your mark somewhere . . . anywhere . . . but there are much better ways to make your mark than garbaging up the world. For instance, you can use the power of protest, financially as well as physically and boycott known polluters to remind them when they trash our world, it is not "GONE WITH THE WIND" and, frankly my dears, WE DO GIVE A DAMN!

CHAPTER 14
Exercise

We exercise because we want to keep in shape or get in shape and exercise does assist us in that area by getting the blood pumping through the capillaries thereby bringing oxygen to the cells. Getting a rapid pulse insures good circulation and keeps the body in proper working order to delay aging and wrinkles. But I believe the real secret to making exercise beneficial is to do something you enjoy. However, before doing any exercise have your doctor check your blood pressure, pulse rate and heart and then start exercising slowly doing a little more each day. Exercise increases the HDL level of the body. That's good cholesterol!

Some wonderfully rewarding body exercises are running, walking, swimming, bicycling, tennis and golf (golf is more beneficial if you don't use a cart, but instead walk the greens). Any of these exercises should be done about 30 minutes a day to get the pulse rate up. Be consistent, don't exercise one week and not the next. If you decide to do it every other day then stick to that.

A friend who runs repeats to himself what he calls his "Running Mantra," "A mile a day keeps the doctor away." Ironically, he is a doctor.

It would be wonderful if every city planner would think to put bicycle paths around town so people could have the option of bicycling instead of driving. Bicycling helps in two ways, it stops pollution and it pumps oxygen into our bodies everytime we pump those pedals. While we're pumping, every body cell is being rejuvenated. The benefits from bicycling are really far reaching. We can lessen pollution, we can become healthier and we can tell OPEC what to do with their oil.

Two things can help make bicycling work for everyone. First we have that all important positive mental attitude, the other is influencing the people in power either personally or in writing to get us good bike paths as alternative transportation.

If you think you can't do it alone just remember someone like Margaret Sanger, the courageous woman who singlehandedly brought birth control information to America with her crusade to change the unjust law against it. The motto she lived by was, "Don't leave the world until you've made it a better place to live in."

However, if you do not get any response for all your efforts and you feel angry and frustrated to the point of causing lines in your face then try the ancient exercise of India: YOGA.

People who practice Yoga know how to turn anger and stress into happiness and relaxation just by proper breathing. One exercise Yogi's do is called the "Breath of Fire." This is a series of short rapid bursts of breath, like an animal panting but the mouth is closed. This sends blood and oxygen racing through your body giving you a natural high. This is a Mother Nature high and is better than anything you can get out of a bottle or from sniffing, snorting or smoking funny grass. Fifty breaths and you feel like you're floating on air. Some people do "Breath of Fire" just before practicing meditation. It brings them up and out of their physical bodies to a more mental and spiritual plane.

Remember, every cell in your body has a rhythm it dances to and it gets energy for this rhythm from oxygen. Try to get extra oxygen into your body everyday, either by exercising or practicing Yoga enough to feel a happy exhilaration because when that happens along comes a positive mental attitude. Then it is much easier to psyche yourself into not being destructive with your body, into staying full of enthusiasm with happiness enough to share with whomever you happen to come in contact.

One exercise that I love is roving. Roving is a combination of running, walking, jogging, skipping and strolling. When I do a mile of this in the morning it gives me a chance to stop and smell the flowers. Some of my friends brag about doing 4 or 5 miles a day and I say, "Wonderful." But I don't try to compete because I'm happier running in my own race. When I tried to do more, I got discouraged and didn't do any.

A simple exercise that I call the lazy man's way to looking better is one that most people overlook. Just turn yourself upside down for 5 minutes a day. It is a proven fact that gravitational forces pull us down every day so I say if you can't beat them, join them. Turn yourself upside down and have gravity work for you instead of against you. Standing on your head can be very easy with a bit of help from a Porta-Yoga. This is a padded stepping stool with the center cut out so your head can hang down while your weight rests on your shoulders. If you can do this 5 minutes in the morning and 5 a night that is even better.

But if you absolutely cannot turn yourself around then lay on a slant board with your feet higher than your head for at least 15 minutes a day, more if you like. This gets the blood into the face and neck area and is an excellent time to do both body and facial exercises. Slant board exercises are also beneficial to relieve congestion about the shoulders, i.e., sinus, weak eyes, falling hair and even ear conditions.

An excellent slant board exercise that forces blood into our heads is to hold on to the sides of the board and bring the knees up to the chest. This also pushes up the abdominal organs if the large intestine is hanging a bit too low from lack of muscle tone. Often this is a problem after childbirth. While in this position turn the head from side to side a few times squeezing the eyes open and shut. Then Air-Bicycle about 20 times. That's the warm up, now there are some basic facial exercises that should be practiced a few times daily.

For that delicate area around the eyes that lines

up first because it is without oil glands try lifting the muscle under the eye back toward the temple without moving eyebrows much. Then lift the area under the eye half way up the eye and relax after a count of 6. Repeat 6 times. The trick is not to let our eyebrows pull the muscle up or your mouth area to push it up. With a bit of concentration and practice you can make the muscle work in a direction that it does not usually go. Use the same idea on other areas of the face and neck that need toning. Try to make the muscle work opposite of the way it usually does. Even doing this just 2 or 3 times every day helps.

Of course, there are areas of the face where lines should be. Laugh lines are nothing to be ashamed of and as Lauren Bacall once said, "Don't retouch my wrinkles, I earned every one of them." That attitude shows self-satisfaction and helps us to "grow old gracefully."

However, most people do not know what that famous cliche really means and how to accomplish it. Growing old gracefully does not mean deep wrinkles and craggy crevices. Part of accomplishing this rare talent is keeping your morale up when you look in the mirror. That is why facial exercises and everything else in this condensed book are very important to you.

The few basic facial exercises I recommend can be done while watching TV or while driving your car. A woman friend of mine used to do facial exercises while driving down the freeway. She said the best part was when other drivers noticed her contortions and just cleared a path so she could drive right on through. She laughed, "Sometimes, when people think you're crazy it has marvelous fringe benefits."

She made facial exercises fun and of course making things fun is another wrinkle eraser. Above all else in life keep your sense of humor. People who don't have a sense of humor age very quickly.

The oldest practicing doctor in the world, Dr. Walter Pannell, age 100, was quoted in a newspaper article as saying, "Stay active and exercise. Not just your body but your mind as well. Then you too can live to be 100."

And actress Mitzi Gaynor, who's now in the second half of 100 and looking great says, "I exercise all the time. My dancing is not enough. I have a full gym at home." To keep the chin line firm she advised isometric exercises. Let your chin rest on your fist then open your mouth while at the same time resisting the jaw's downward movement with your fist. Do 10 times a day. She also recommend wiggling your ears 200 times a day but so far I haven't managed that fete.

I do a couple of easy exercises for better under the chin muscle tone. One is just keeping your mouth shut and pressing your tongue against the back of your bottom teeth or against the roof of your mouth for a count of six. The other is pulling your head back and pushing your lower lip over your top lip for a five count then consciously lift the chin muscles up for another 5 count. Repeat 6 times a day.

COLOR, MUSIC & YOGA

Most people don't think about the simple things in life that keep us well like the color we might see during a day or night, the music we might hear and the bending and stretching of our muscles.

Science tells us that color is vibration of light,

light is radiant energy. Color enters through our eyes and has an immediate reaction on our physical, emotional, mental and even our spiritual feelings. It is vitally important to have colors in our homes that are pleasing to our senses. If they are not, then redecorating isn't a luxury it is a necessity for our well being.

As we go through life we may find that colors we have lived with for a long time are not emotionally satisfying anymore. In other words, we are bored with them and it's time for a change to give us a fresh new feeling which almost always gives us more joy in living.

Our first preference for a certain color may start right in the cradle. I know that with my twin daughters I put one in a pink basinette and the other in yellow and to this day the one that was in pink prefers pink and the one that was in yellow prefers yellow.

But going back to basics, our genetic coloring often helps us to choose colors we prefer because a certain color may look better with green eyes, or blonde hair or dark skin.

Most of us have had a friend greet us at one time or another with, "Hey that color looks great on you." And often other people will react to you in a more receptive way if your color combination is appealing. And you will react in a more favorable way because you feel good about the way you look.

Whenever I walk I always take the time to enjoy the colors that may be blossoming on some tree, or may be painted on some house or building or may be worn by a passing person. This may very well be what is meant by, "The best things in life are free."

The things that enter into our psyche through our senses that make us feel better because we personally enjoy them.

This of course, is true about music also. Nobody understands the power of music better than governments. They have often used marching music to inspire men to go to war. And the people who make motion pictures use music to set a mood. An audience can be scared right out of their seats just from the spooky music in a melodrama.

During the 60's and 70's parents blamed rock and then acid rock for the drug culture, the weird clothing and the bizarre behavior of their offsprings.

Traditionally waltzes and classical music are used to soothe the savage beast in us. And the big bands of the 40's played music that just made us feel good about ourselves. And now in the 90's we find the 40's music is being revived because we need to just feel good about ourselves again. And feeling good about ourselves definitely helps us to stay well and happy.

But a few more words on facial exercises before going to the next step in my 5 point plant. When doing facial exercises be sure to remove all makeup and leave a light moisturizer on the face. I don't believe it's necessary to put a heavy, thick cream over the skin. I believe it suffocates the pores and the whole body breathes through the pores.

Start every exercise by relaxing your throat and facial muscles and letting your head drop forward and roll it completely around to the right then to the left about 3 times. Lift your shoulders up to your ears and let them drop about 5 times. Then stand with your feet apart so your body is equally balanced on both feet and swing your right arm around 30 times, do the same with your left arm. This is a good way to get the blood pumping above the waist so when you do your facial exercises they are twice as effective as they would be if you were sedentary. Lack of circulation causes muscular atrophy, of course that causes wrinkles.

For the next exercises you can sit down in front of a mirror but remember when seated not to slouch. The upper lip is another area vulnerable to lines and wrinkling. Open your mouth and move the upper lip down over the front teeth then slowly pull it back up again. Repeat 6 times. Here again the idea is to move the muscle in the opposite direction of normal movement. Usually these muscles are pulled sideways when we smile but rarely are they pulled forward and down unless we pucker up to whistle but with this exercise you don't want to pucker.

The best part about Yoga or any bending and stretching exercise is that it basically helps our bodies to stay limber thereby keeping our circulation in good working condition. Circulation is helped by breathing properly and Yoga teaches us the importance of proper inhaling and exhaling. That's why I prefer it to the more strenuous aerobic type of exercises. I tried those aerobic classes but I'm afraid that I qualify as a Jane Fonda reject, a dyslexic aerobic. I never seemed to be jumping in synch with the rest of the class. So I have to find my own form of exercise. Which as I have said is quite often just hanging around upside down or resting on a slant board.

ACUPUNCTURE

Lately acupuncture has come into popularity as a way to face lifting. I have tried it and found it beneficial in that it stimulates the circulation under the skin therefore I feel it should be included in this chapter on facial exercise.

When I wanted to find out more about acupuncture I went to Dr. R. Uy, M.D., a woman physician and surgeon in Los Angeles who was also trained in China as an acupuncture specialist.

Acupuncture therapy was established about 4,000 years ago in China. This art of healing by acupuncture represents the slow accumulation of experience by many practitioners. The earliest documentation is found in The Cannon of Medicine, a Chinese medical treatise, compiled about 2,400 years back. It contains a description of the anatomical locations of acupuncture points, of mental and physical disorders, and methods of therapy. It also contains a chart of the meridian system, the theory that underlies all acupuncture practice.

California leads the country in the number of qualified acupuncturists. Although an acupuncturist may have practised the art in China, he or she is still required to be licensed in California by the State Board of Medical Quality Assurance. To obtain the license, an acupuncturist must have had at least 5 years of acupuncture training and pass a state written, oral land clinical exam.

For face lifting help Dr. Uy recommends 10 to 12 treatments and a booster treatment every 3 months. I had 10 treatments and as I said the basic benefit is the stimulation of circulation under the skin thereby helping the skin to retain its elasticity and to help in cell regeneration.

A side benefit is the relaxation one feels after the needles are inserted and you rest for half an hour to forty-five minutes. Acupuncture also works on the body as an anesthetic by releasing endorphins.

Endorphins are a group of hormone-like protein substances produced in the brain following acupuncture therapy. These substances negate pain sensations and encourage other biochemical functions such as the production of white blood cells to fight infections.

Using acupuncture for face lifting is not the way to get a dramatic instant face lift as one might expect from plastic surgery. It is a more gradual benefit but it also does not have the potential risk that goes with any surgery. I am not against plastic surgery. I just believe in looking good as long as possible without surgery. If you can look good into your fifties without surgery, great! But when surgery is necessary then go for it. After surgery rejuvenate with vegetable juices preferably made fresh with your own juicer.

CHAPTER 15
Crack A Smile, Not Your Skin

How much do you know about the care and feeding of the outer layer of your skin? We are all bombarded with information from cosmetics companies on how to care for our skin but they never tell us you really have to start with the inner to get to the outer. Your body talks to you from the inside out. Often when you get a headache it is a warning signal that the body is clogged somewhere and your chemical balance is off. Then that's the time to not take an aspirin but take an enema or a laxative to clean out the problem. When you feel better, you look better. And it always helps to start from the ground up.

Shoes! Sometimes I think the shoe manufacturers must be paid by the foot doctors and the cosmetic companies to give women foot trouble. Pointed toe, stilt high heels are the first step women take towards foot problems. And if you have sore feet you'll be frowning and causing wrinkles in the face and all from those expensive shoes that are such high style.

Personally I'll take comfort over what's in style any day. I find it more fun to create my own style.

Now, when you feel better, there are some basic foods that help to keep you looking better. The top ten are legumes, spinach, raw skim milk, garlic, broccoli, strawberries, whole grains, turkey, fish and tofu.

Garlic is rich in sulfur needed for healthy skin, nails and hair. Legumes include, lentils, split peas, pinto beans, chick peas and most green vegetables because they contain B vitamins to help keep blood circulating for that glowing look. Spinach has iron and a supply of A and C vitamins. Raw skim milk has calcium and Broccoli contains Vitamin A which is necessary to maintain skin structure and renew cells. It also has vitamin C which promotes healthy skin and gums. The fiber in these vegetables helps keep the digestive system moving along smoothly. Turkey only has 55 calories per oz., is full of B vitamins and potassium and is just as low in fat as fish. Whole grains help maintain skin elasticity and fish has most of the B vitamins including B 12 and protein. Tofu, a soybean curd, is high in calcium which prevents bone deterioration. It has protein but the protein is not complete and should be supplemented with rice or grains.

All natural foods are better for your body and your looks than man-made processed foods. Try to eat a varied diet which includes foods you're not crazy about because if you eat only foods you like all the time you could develop an allergy to one or more simply from over use. If you feel you have developed an allergy to a particular food stop eating it for one or two months and try it again. In other words, let the body take a break from it for awhile.

Now what about skin moisturizers and all the claims we hear about collagen and elastin creams. Collagen and elastin molecules in creams are too large and heavy to penetrate beneath the skin's superficial layers. They remain on the surface, sealing in water like any ordinary moisturizer.This may make wrinkles less obvious but there is no evidence externally applied collagen and elastin creams can replenish the skin's natural collagen and elastin fibers. Moisturizers help wrinkles by keeping the skin moist and the best time to apply them is when the skin is moist. Spraying it with a fine water mist is good but if you don't have a spritzer then splash water on, pat half dry and apply moisturizer. As we get more mature, our skin tends to produce less oil so it is essential that some kind of cream protection be used.

Moisturizing needs are different for different skin types. However, usually light creams are better because heavy creams can clog pores. As for most touted eye creams they are too greasy. There is no need to buy several different expensive creams. A good moisturizing cream can be used on the face, eye area and neck. It is true that most of the time you get what you pay for and the more expensive item is many times better, however, when it comes to cosmetics this old truism is no longer true. In fact, some very expensive cosmetics could be more harmful than the less expensive. A well-known model found this out the hard way and wound up suing the Erno Laszlo Institute for two million dollars because after spending more than $400 for Laszlo products her skin broke out and became scarred for life. Not only was her career destroyed but her marriage broke up from the pain, suffering and emotional stress. Obviously Laszlo cosmetics have not affected everyone this way or they would be out of business.

When trying a new cream or cosmetic it is wise to buy a small amount or to get samples and try them first. Moisturizers contain different fragrances and preservatives and you may be allergic to one of these substances. An allergy can appear on the skin as redness, itching, a rash or pimples.

What about sunscreens? If you are going to be out in the sun for more than 20 minutes then use a sunscreen cream, but the stronger the sunscreen the more likely a person could develop an allergy to it. Again one must test what is best for their own skin.

Besides wearing a makeup base with a sunscreen I wear a hat with a visor or wide brim and sunglasses. And, a word of caution about perfumes and/or hairsprays. Be careful not to get them on the face because the sun can cause a permanent brown spot on your skin when it penetrates the perfume or spray. The most intense sun is between the hours of 11 a.m. and 3 p.m.

There are some beauticians who say never use soap on the face but these days there are so many different types of soaps that that statement no longer is true. There are cold cream, oatmeal, olive oil and lemon soaps to name just a few. Again I say experiment to find what is best for you. I alternate between cleansing creams and soaps. Some nights my skin feels drier than others then I use a cream. There are soap substitute cleansers such as Cetaphil and the Metrin company makes an excellent cleanser and moisturizer. Also Complex 15 is a good light moisturizer. I am usually allergic to most eye make-up removers but I have found that Lancome's Effacil eye makeup remover works best for me and I don't get my usual eye rashes from it.

I also use Albolene, Noxema, an oatmeal soap and a lemon scented soap I get at health food stores. There are an abundance of creams and cleansers but only you can really know what is good for your particular skin.

Chlorophyll is a good deodorant for the body and also brings oxygen to the cells. All green vegetables contain chlorophyll. You can also get it at most health food stores either bottled or in the form of wheat grass but remember not to over do, too much concentrated chlorophyll can cause vomiting.

No matter what you do fair skin will age quicker than dark skin. Wherever the temperature is hot, the skin color is normally dark, the further towards the north pole one lives the lighter the skin. This proves that skin color is precisely a function of the weather and evolution. Darker skin has melanin, a dark pigment that helps to protect the skin against the ravages of the sun. However, dark skin people should use moisturizers also because there are other factors that dry out the skin besides the sun, i.e. excess salt or alcohol, not drinking enough water (usually a minimum of 6 glasses a day) and smoking.

From the cradle thru the "golden years" moisturizing is necessary. Recently a friend I hadn't seen in a few years said I looked the same. Yes, I thought, it just takes me longer. The years will make a difference no matter how good we might take care of ourselves but the object is to make it a gradual difference, to grow old gracefully. This is not to say that if one feels a face lift is necessary they shouldn't have one. I say, whatever makes you feel and look better is worth doing.

When we do have wrinkles there are a few, makeup tricks that can be used. For crepey eyelids use a moisturizer undercoat before applying eye shadow and never use iridescent shadow. For wrinkles around the eye area beauty expert, Rachel Perry, says they can be camouflaged with a cream lighter than your skin then cover it with your makeup base. Also for hard to hide wrinkles use a light colored eye shadow, white or very light beige in the deepest part of the wrinkle, put it on before you put on powder and it will last all day.

I do not think the face should be touched anymore than is absolutely necessary because it is too easy to stretch delicate facial skin. Therefore I do not believe frequent facials are beneficial. If the average person uses a facial scrub once a month that should be sufficient after 40. Soap should be kept to once a week and then it should be a special face soap that won't dry out the skin. Here again trying a few different types for your particular face is the only way to find out which one is suited to your skin type.

On a daily basis I usually clean my face with a good cold pressed natural oil such as Olive, Safflower, Sesame, Almond or Jojoba. Sometimes I mix this with Ponds cold creme or Albolene to get a little thicker consistency.

The Jojoba plant is native to the southern California desert and is reputed to be beneficial to both skin and hair.

When I remove my make-up I make faces while applying the oil and while wiping it off with an old terry cloth towel. I think terry towel is better and easier on the skin than tissue which comes from the bark of a tree. I also like some liquid facial soaps but again I say experiment and find whats best for your type of skin.

During the day I use a light moisturizer, preferably made with PABA and natural ingredients and no perfumes. I am an avid label reader and I look for natural products not only when I buy food but when I buy facial and body creams as well. Some ingredients I've found beneficial are lecithin, PABA, cucucumber, wheat germ, soy protein and chamomile. However, some people are even allergic to natural products like Paba or Aloe Vera.

Chamomile is especially helpful to me when my skin gets hives or just blotchy red. I have what is known as "English Skin" coming from ancestors who sailed across the English channel on Viking ships from Denmark. My roots have been traced back to King Canute, a Danish Viking who managed to conquer Ethelred the Unready and become the first King of England. Lucky for him that Ethelred was unready but unlucky for me that I inherited a redheads sensitive skin. I tell you this to prove I was not born with a tough hide but with very delicate skin and it is not my ancestry that keeps my wrinkles at bay, it is really my determination and my five point plan.

Sometimes when my skin gets especially irritated from too much sun or smog or indulging in some food or drink I shouldn't have then I make Chamomile tea, let it cool and pat it on my face with a ball of cotton. Then I'll drink what's left, this has a soothing effect. Also pure Aloe Vera Gel is excellent to tame the red Dragon as I call it. In fact, Aloe has been known to cure ulcers when taken internally. As little as a tablespoon a day helps.

Recently a newspaper article proclaimed, "Amazing Vitamin Cream Makes Aged Skin Look Young Again." Then they went on to say it was a face lift in a tube. Well this so-called miracle cream could do more damage than help. Retinoic Acid does have Vitamin A in it among other ingredients but what it does is peel off the top layer of skin. When you use it you'll notice a slight redness which increases until the outer skin peels off, usually within 36 hours.

However, when I talked with Dr. James Fulton, Jr., an acne specialist, about this he did not believe that it helps to delay wrinkles, in fact he believed it could very well put more wrinkles in the skin than were originally there. When using Retinoic Acid it is absolutely a must to stay out of the sun for at least 10 days but if the sun does hit the skin it will wrinkle more than before because the skin has become thinner.

Dr. Fulton also believes that Dermabrasion is better than a chemical peel if one is considering that type of process to regain a youthful appearance. It takes 12 chemicals peels to equal 1 dermabrasion and chemical peels can be very painful plus theoretically there is no way of controlling just how deep the chemical will penetrate into the skin. I also believe in face lifts when the skin has lost its elasticity. As Dolly Parton said when asked if she'd ever had plastic surgery. "I think most of us have had as many lifts as a naked hitchhiker!" which fits into my basic motto: "Whatever works!" to make us feel good about ourselves. I just don't believe in having it before you really need it because surgery of any kind puts stress on the body. Many women have peels and plastic surgery before fifty. This book helps one to look better longer and hopefully to delay the surgery stress until after 50.

I'm sure by now most people know how damaging the sun can be to human skin. Sun dries and wrinkles even the youngest skin especially if exposure is more than an hour, so moisturizers are definitely necessary. A good moisturizer should contain a sunscreen and usually that means using PABA. PABA is a member of the B complex family and it helps to prevent exzema and loss of pigmentation. It has vital sunscreening properties as does another ingredient used in many sunscreening moisturizers called Octyl Dimethyl. Everyone out in the sun squints aginst its rays, so using a good moisturizer around the eye area will help delay wrinkles that are not laugh lines.

Many people involved in the health field, i.e., Doctors, Nutritionists and the multitudes who advise avoiding saturated fats and using more polyunsaturated fats are trying to be helpful. I do not totally agree with this. Tests have shown that polyunsaturated fats speed up the skin's aging because the vitamins and minerals that help to prevent the skins aging have been taken out of this refined product.

Therefore, I reiterate what I have said pre-

viously about natural foods even in the fat department. If you are going to eat fats then eat natural fats
but just eat them in smaller quantities. It really isn't
that butter or natural whipped cream are bad for you
it is more that most people who like these foods eat
too much at one time.

OILS

Have you checked your oil lately! Years ago all
seed or animal fat sources were prepared by mechanical processing without heat — cold processing. In
many countries even today, major vegetable oils are
still prepared simply by cleaning and pressing the
sources, thus producing clean but unrefined oils.

Contrast this to the Americanization of vegetable oils and you will see what we have done to fats —
what in the past we did to sugars and flours.
(Stripped them of Mother Nature's nutritional
packaging).

The process to which we subject oils always
deteriorates their nutritional and health quality, and
never improves it. Since fats are used both in the
structure of our cells and the metabolism, then
altered fats can damage both our cells and our metabolism. Processed oils reduce nutritional value of
oils in the following ways:

1. The amount of polyunsaturated fatty acids,
   especially linolenic acid is reduced drastically.

2. Refining removes significant amounts of the
   vitamins that are a part of the original fat rich
   food sources.

   Vitamin A is cut down severely as is Vitamin C.
   Oil seeds contain significant amount of minerals
   and trace elements, processing eliminates these

almost entirely.

3. Plant sterols are removed, these are "good" relatives of cholesterol and resemble it so much that they fit into the gates through which cholesterol would otherwise enter, blocking its entrance into the blood.

4. Lecithins are eliminated. This is unfortunate because Lecithins are involved in the function of an enzyme called LCAT (Lecithin-cholesterol acyl transferase). LCAT is the biochemical hero that actually helps remove cholesterol deposits from within blood vessels.

5. The high temperatures that are used in modern oil processing also tend to form new hybrid molecules. Some of these by-products have not been studied carefully enough so there is no assurance of their safety.

Production methods of commercial processed vegetable oils require that the oils be dissolved in a chemical, usually hexane. This mixture is then heated thus separating the oil from the hexane (allowing the hexane to be recycled). Typically the next step in the refining process uses caustic soda or soda ash and phosphoric acid. Next, the oil is bleached with acid treated diatomaceous earth and sometimes with charcoal. Deodorizing is usually accomplished by using live steam at temperatures of 400-470° for 1 to 2 hours.

If the oils are to be hydrogenated the process then uses heat, pressure and a small amount of nickel, to force hydrogen into the molecules of the oil. This destroys the double bonds of the fat and saturates them.

On a positive note, the advantages of conventionally processed oils are: a) extends shelf life dramatically; b) removes impurities and pesticides that may be present in the seeds.

The problem is to find a true source of wholesome, nutritionally rich oil, hygenically processed, and manufactured in a light and air free environment. The oil should then be packaged in dark glass containers for optimum protection. The solution to finding the perfect oil is FLORA'S OILS.

FLORA'S Oils are unique in that they are freshly cold processed, unrefined, non-deodorized, unfiltered, with nothing taken away or added.

FLORA'S Oils are excellent in lowering blood cholesterol and they are high in Linoleic and Linolenic acid.

FLORA'S Oils are rich and tasty . . . so flavorful . . . they bring out the essence of the seeds themselves. Their exquisite taste is a gourmet's delight.

The oils have a shelf life of approximately 3 to 3½ months. These oils have been used successfully by Dr. Johanna Budwick, of Germany, in her treatment of degenerative diseases.

Presently, the oils are produced by Flora Manufacturing, 7400 Fraser Park Drive, Burnaby, BC, V5J B59, Canada. (604) 438-1133. Flora has 12 different varieties of oil — most of them certified organic. Flora's oils are sold in Canada at the local health store.

Flora oils are available in the U.S.A. Their address is 805 E. Badger, Lynden, WA. 98264, (206) 354-2110.

Flora oils are an excellent source of essential fatty acids and help build the immune system.

The best and most healthful oils for the human body are Olive, Flax or Linseed, Safflower, Sunflower and Corn and all of these should be pure cold-pressed because the body assimilates them more efficiently. All oils in moderation can be safe but studies show that saturated fats raise blood cholesterol levels. Generally, the higher the percentage of unsaturated fats the healthier the oil.

Oils, such as corn oils are made up mostly of polyunsaturated fats which lower overall blood cholesterol. Oils such as Olive oil are made up mostly of monounsaturated fats, found by some researchers to lower levels of low-density/lipoproteins (LDLs). Low-density lipoproteins are the bad type of cholesterol. High density lipoproteins (HDL's) are the good type of cholesterol believed to protect against cholesterol deposits within blood vessels.

As has been stated polyunsaturated fats are not risk free and should not be used excessively. Ingesting large amounts of salad and cooking oils and other largely polyunsaturated fats has also been associated with gallstones. In animal studies, high levels of polyunsaturated fats have been associated with potential suppression of the immune system and some forms of cancer. And even though polyunsaturated fats reduce total blood cholesterol, high levels of polyunsaturated fats can lower HDL "good" cholesterol.

Oils that are very high in saturated fats are Cottonseed oil, Palm Kernal Oil and Coconut oil. Saturated vegetables oils will raise blood cholesterol higher than beef fat, butter or lard.

Oils should be stored in cold areas such as a cold pantry or a refrigerator. Oils oxidize easily and get rancid but Olive oil will solidify if refrigerated and should be taken out about thirty minutes before usage.

Partially hydrogenated is a phrase often used on labels and it means that the fat has been made more saturated through processing. Hydrogenation increases the shelf life, which is good for the manufacturer's profits but not good for the consumer's health. Some labels may read, "Contains one of the following" and they list several oils which may or may not be in the product. This is also a convenience for the manufacturer. They want to be able to change an oil without relabeling, depending on supply and demand and cost . . . not necessarily in that order.

Consumers are often drawn to labels that read "Cholesterol-free." This is misleading since none of the oils contains cholesterol. When a label says "Cholesterol-free" it does not mean fat-free. Oils are all 100% fat.

The following chart compares vegetables oils:

COMPARING VEGETABLE OILS

Fatty Acid Content

Type	Percent Polyun-saturated	Percent Monoun-saturated	Percent saturated	Unsaturated/ Saturated Fat Ratio	Comment
Canola*	32	62	6	15:7:1	Best fatty acid ratio.
Safflower	75	12	9	9.6:1	Highest in polyunsaturates.
Sunflower	66	20	10	8.6:1	Sometimes used in place of olive oil,but blander.
Corn	59	24	13	6.4:1	Heavy taste. Often used for deep frying.
Soybean	59	23	14	5.9:1	Most commonly used oil — in baked goods, salad dressings, margarine, mayonnaise.
Olive	9	72	14	5.8:1	Highest in monounsaturated fat. Expensive.
Peanut	32	46	17	4.6:1	More pronounced flavor than most oils.
Sesame seed	40	40	18	4.4:1	Used in Oriental and Middle Eastern cooking.Flavorful.
Cottonseed	52	18	26	2.7:1	Comparatively high in saturated fat. Used in processed foods, salad dressings.
Palm kernel	2	10	80	0.2:1	The only vegetable oils high in saturated fat. Used in
Coconut	2	6	87	0.1:1	baked goods and candies.

*an oil made from a turnip-like plant.

Note: Other substances, such as water and vitamins, make up the total composition (100%)
Adapted from UC Berkeley Wellness Letter, March, 1987.

In a book entitled, *Sunlight Could Save Your Life,* by Dr. Zane R. Kime, MD, MS, he writes about the problem of polyunsaturated fats accelerating skin aging in Chapter 4, "Sunlight and Aging." Dr. Kime says, "Only in the last few decades has the accelerated aging of the skin become so noticeable especially since Americans have increased their intake of polyunsaturated fat." He goes on to explain that some of the culprits to aging are "free radical formation" which is the phenomena that happens whan fat oils turn rancid when exposed to air. Certain vitamins and minerals that prevent free radical formation are found in abundance in the natural foodstuffs. These are removed when food is refined."

Thank you Dr. Kime for confirming what I already suspected, even before I studied for my Master of Science degree.

If you suffer from skin problems like acne, psoriasis, eczema, and a general excess of pimples it just may be your're getting too much protein. Americans have a tendency to overdose on proteins and an overabundance can cause internal toxins that rise up to plague our skin. But it's not just the meat eaters who have this problem, vegetarians who consume too many nuts, cheeses, eggs and other dairy products can also be vexed by this annoying problem.

We are taught that protein builds cells but they usually fail to add that a very small amount is needed, on an average less than half an ounce at a meal. Even an ounce a day is sufficient and people have survived quite nicely on only 3 to 4 ounces a week.

Actress and health food advocate the late Gloria Swanson told a story about herself regarding protein that is quite interesting. When she was very young, thirty was very young to Gloria, she developed a tumor and her medical doctor wanted to operate to perform a hysterectomy thereby getting rid of the tumor and a few other incidentals. Fortunately, Gloria had read a book called *Food Is Your Best Medicine* by Dr. Henry Bieler, M.D. and she went to see Dr. Bieler. After reviewing her diet he told her she had overdone protein and built her own tumor. He advised cutting down on her protein intake and then in his opinion her tumor just might dissolve of its own accord. As crazy as this sounded to her at the time it didn't sound as crazy as getting a hysterectomy so she decided to give it a try. It took two years to completely disappear but she followed his instructions and never did have the hysterectomy. She told her old doctor what had happened and refused to pay his bill. He accepted her refusal. And Gloria, even in her eighties, had beautiful clear skin.

On the opposite end of getting enough exercise is getting enough rest and sleep. When the body is exhausted, nothing can rejuvenate it but a good nights sleep. Rest and sleep are another personal area. Some people feel fine and look great with just 5 or 6 hours of sleep while others not only require the full 8 hours at night but also a little mini-nap during the afternoon is necessary. A mini-nap could be anywhere from 20 minutes to an hour.

At night I sleep with my feet slightly elevated. As I have said, gravity is constantly pulling us down so we have to fight back. When we reverse our position we get gravity working for us instead of against us. You can elevate your feet by putting a couple of pillows under them or buy a foam rubber pad or if you feel like splurging on yourself buy an electric bed that lifts up at both ends like the kind hospitals use.

It seems that nature has designed us to sleep when it's dark and wake when it's light. Generally this works very well in helping us to look and feel our best. Many doctors advocate getting a full 8 hours sleep at night but Dr. James E. Fulton, Jr., a specialist in skin care, believes that the body rejuvenates itself best when sleeping between the hours of 11 p.m. and 7 a.m. Dr. Fulton operates several acne skin care clinics and he says a loss of sleep on a chronic basis can leave permanent wrinkles in the face. He stressed to me what he calls the three S-s for beautiful skin — sleep, no smoking and sunscreens. If you really want to delay those wrinkles it is vitally important to get enough sleep, between the right hours, to use a sunscreen outdoors if you're under the sun for any length of time, and of course not to smoke anything, as any kind of smoke cuts off vital oxygen to the cells.

Dr. Arnold Fox, MD, author of "The Beverly Hills Medical Diet" and a nutrition minded physician who specializes in internal and preventive medicine explained, when I interviewed him, about the process of the body's circadian rhythms. Circadian rhythms are the normal ebb and flow of the body's hormones. The normal flow of our adrenal hormones is very low between the hours of 3 and 6 a.m. The sleep we get at this time is very important to revitalizing the entire body. He said Dr. Charles Stroble, a Psychiatrist and Bio-feedback specialist at Harvard, found out a great deal about our circadian rhythms from tests he conducted. The main thing he learned from his tests was that when our adrenal hormones are low we are generally depleted of energy. The usual hours for this depletion are between midnight and before 6 a.m. Accordingly, this would be the best time to be asleep.

If not asleep then hopefully you are not having a great deal of stress at those hours. If you work nights it should be a job you enjoy. Even if you're asleep at that time you could be having a stressful nightmare and people have been known to have heart attacks in their sleep.

Dr. Fox agreed with me that the average physician is not trained in the science of nutrition and usually knows very little about the main thing that keeps the body in good shape. What is mainly taught at most medical schools is surgery and drugs. He said something I've rarely heard from a man of medicine, "There is one vital area that most doctors overlook and that is the power of the mind to make us well. Personally, I would rather give a prayer than a prescription."

All I can add to that is Amen.

While we are on the subject of sleep I would like to mention sleeping positions. The best way to avoid facial wrinkles is to sleep on your back. If you must use a pillow then use it under the back of your neck and not in a position where it pushes lines into your face. You might think that those lines wear off after a few hours but if you sleep squashing your face in the same way night after night those lines will become indelible. Then, even if your body feels rejuvenated after a good nights rest your face won't reflect all of that rejuvenation.

Almost in the same area as rest and sleep is Meditation. Many wonderful things have been said about meditation. It has helped people cope with everyday problems and it has kept others from having nervous breakdowns. Although I have never heard it said by anyone else that meditation keeps wrinkles away I believe it does help. Even if it just takes a worried look off your face it's a step in the right direction.

Meditation has been known to slow down the pulse rate, lift the mind to an altered state of consciousness; almost like a dream state and to lower the body temperature. We all know that lowering temperatures preserves meat so all this would be beneficial to the body as well as the mind.

Nutritionist, author Gayelord Hauser, who died at 89, once told me, "When I pray I talk to God, ah, but when I meditate I listen to God."

Over the years it has been my observation that a truly youthful, vibrant appearance does not seem to stay with most people who are totally involved with the materialistic world and have no spiritual values whatsoever. Rather than go into a long dissertation on this I will quote one meditation prayer that for me sums it all up.

"Lord make me an instrument of thy peace
Where there is hatred, let me sow love
Where there is injury, pardon,
Where there is despair, hope,
Where there is doubt, faith,
Where there is darkness, light,
Where there is sadness, joy.
O Divine Master, grant that I may not so much
     seek to be consoled as to console,
To be understood as to understand,
To be loved as to love,
For it is in giving that we receive
It is in pardoning that we are pardoned,
It is dying (to self) that we are born to eternal
     life."

I try to take 15 minutes a day where I close my eyes, blank out my mind, inhale 25 or more deep relaxing breaths and meditate. Do this in a comfortable position. Some people sit on the floor with their legs crossed and their back straight. I prefer my legs tucked under my buttocks and my feet resting on a pillow so they are slightly elevated behind me.

When you first start to meditate you might want

to set a timer so you'll know when 15 minutes are over. After you've meditated for awhile you will automatically know when your meditation period is over.

Hopefully meditation will leave you feeling satisfied and serene . . . not an easy task these days.

PLANT ENZYMES

The National Enzyme Company was started by Dr. Edward Howell in the 1930's for the purpose of conducting research and development of food enzyme supplements. The Food Enzyme Concept, as described in his two books, Enzyme Nutrition and Food Enzymes for Health and Longevity basically points out that all cooked and processed foods have lost their naturally occurring food enzymes. The enzymes normally associated with each raw food in its natural state is the correct balance to digest those foods.

The destruction of the food enzymes (through the cooking process) leads to an increase of stress on the digestive system of man to produce digestive enzymes to do the work which should have been done by the food enzymes in the upper stomach. This stress leads to organ hyperthrophy, eventual organ breakdown and incomplete or inefficient assimilation and utilization of foods, nutrients, supplements etc. By supplementing the food enzymes back in, we can more effectively digest the foods we eat, and thereby make the nutrients more available to the body with less stress on the digestive and immune systems. In addition, this leads to better assimilation and utilization of supplements utilized as well.

FOOD ENZYMES

Doctor Howell's enzyme formulations are available in various forms in the health food industry. Interested parties may write to the International Enzyme Foundation, P.O. Box 2; Wilmont, Wisconsin 53192, Phone No. (414) 862-6968.

These food enzyme supplements have been used successfully by hundreds of thousands of satisfied users over the last 50 years. Doctors and health care professionals recommend these food enzymes enthusiastically.

Their enzymes are 100-percent vegetarian and are superior to all other enzymes, because they can function in both the first and third stages of digestion (and therefore can work throughout the digestive tract). This is crucially important because it is in the first stage of digestion that food enzymes exhibit their greatest activity. The Enzyme Foundation supplements provide all four food enzyme groups that function in this critical digestive stage.

Most enzyme supplements like pepsin, trypsin, papain and bromolain contain only protease enzymes. These enzymes digest proteins, but have no value whatsoever where fats, carbohydrates and cellulose are concerned.

Beneficial enzyme supplements must contain all four enzyme groups, which are: protease for proteins, lipase for fats, carbohydrase for carbohyddrates, and cellulase for cellulose. (These groups are also helpful in digesting protein).

Our body's organs — especially the pancreas — produce enzymes for the purpose of digesting foods, as well as supplying our organs the enzymes they need. It's still vital to get enzymes in the diet because our pancreas and other enzyme-making organs, as well as the metabolic processes of the body, need a chance to rest. This is especially true when organs have been overused in producing enzymes to process refined foods that take away digestive juices and give nothing back to the body's health process.

It may be noted that the dramatic digestive effects can be most easily seen when using plant enzymes to replace the food enzymes, as these enzymes work in the acid environment of the upper stomach, ahead of the body's primary digestive organs, while other types of enzyme supplements, such as pancreatin, only work in the alkaline environment of the small intestine, which does not relieve the stress of digestive activity from the body as the important function of "predigestion" is not accomplished by such pancreatic enzyme supplements.

Nature designed the human body when there were no refined or processed foods and there was a minimum of cooked foods.

Yes, food enzymes may be the missing link to optimum health.

KYOLIC GARLIC/FOOD ENZYMES SUPPLEMENTS FORMULA 102

By combining the well-known values of garlic with the potency of plant enzyme supplementation to replace the missing food enzymes, it is possible to achieve levels of digestion and assimilation not generally seen in modern society, while reducing the stress occurring to the body's own digestive system. Many people have experienced the dramatic dif-

ference possible through garlic/enzyme combina-
tions. Kyolic formula 102 incorporates these plant
enzymes with their renown odorless garlic. Kyolic
formula 102 is a very potent formula and comes in
capsules and tablet forms.

CHAPTER 16
Knowing Yourself

Knowing yourself could very well be the most important part of delaying wrinkles. Because if you are confused about your own identity then worry lines begin to etch themselves across your forehead and around your eyes. A great many people are confused about who they are and what they should do with their lives.

The reason for this is because it usually takes us awhile to get used to ourselves. Sometimes 30 or 40 years and sometimes an entire lifetime. A girlfriend of mine once told me that her whole life was a big question mark and what she wanted written across her tombstone was the simple epitaph: "What Was That All About?" I'm sure we have all felt that way at one time or another.

But if you find at some point that you are not

satisfied with your life then it is time to re-evaluate who you are and what you want from your existence.

Are you doing the things that are satisfying to you? Are you with the people you really like? And if not, why not? Remember, and on this point many psychiatrists and psychologists agree, if you are not honest with yourself you can not be honest with anyone else.

Have you ever seen the look of a self-satisfied person? They seem to have a relaxed aura about them that makes them appear happy and well-adjusted. It doesn't matter what their chronological age is. Their physical appearance always seems younger and other people are attracted to them because of their zest for life. Two celebrities that come to my mind as outstanding examples of this are Douglas Fairbanks, Jr. and Ginger Rogers. They really make the second half of life look like the best half. They wear their years extremely well with a youthful exuburance that is as elusive as the butterfly of love.

I believe the key to this youthfulness is simple. Find your identity and settle in comfortably with it. This does not in any way limit a person's lifestyle. All we have to do is mix a bit of imagination with a little daring and we can lead very exciting and rewarding lives.

The one great asset about living now in the end of the 20th Century is that most of us in a "modern" society can lead any type of lifestyle we like without risking our lives to do so. Needless to say, this keeps worry lines off the face. And the more people who live just the kind of life they want the more accepting society will become. When that happens we can all relax and be more comfortable and our faces will reflect this serenity.

Too many people go through life acting the way other people expect them to, simply because they are fearful of rejection. But in reality, if they stopped to think about it, what they fear the most, rejection, is exactly what they are getting. By hiding their true personality they are not being accepted for themselves and all this weighs heavily on their id. The id is that part of the psyche, constituting the unconscious which is the source of instinctual energy. In other words they just don't have the energy. You can always see this type of exhaustion reflected in the lines on a person's face. They can eat all the health food they need and exercise from dawn till dusk but if they have not found themselves it isn't going to erase those facial lines.

I am often puzzled by the fact that most people are so sure they know what is normal that they condemn anyone else that may think differently. Yet most of the sexual research that has been done from Freud, to Kinsey, to Masters and Johnson tell us that the human being on planet earth can be sexually attracted to almost anything or anyone. We should be more open as to what is naturally human and stop worrying about our sexual natures so much that it causes worry lines on our faces.

I have always believed that the worst poverty on earth is not living in a small room but living in a small mind.

When we do have an intimate knowledge of ourselves we can always improve on some facet of our personaltiy that we do not like. This personal knowledge is like having a basic blueprint of our souls. How nice to be able to work from our foundations on up. It makes us so much easier to live with. When we do not think well of ourselves it's difficult to understand how anyone else can like us. Therefore we make life miserable not only for ourselves but also for the ones around us.

When I was in my 30's I became very critical of myself. I thought I had lost my looks because after having children my figure didn't compare to what it was before these "blessed events." And it certainly didn't match up to what I saw in Playboy magazine. I even rushed out to the nearest plastic surgeons to see what could be done but fortunately I didn't rush to do anything. One night after gathering my information and analyzing my life I rationalized that if someone liked me they would like me even if I were not physically perfect and if they did not like me they wouldn't like me any better if my face and body were perfect.

So I took the first step toward easing the wrinkles in my face by being nice to myself with a little understanding and love. After then it became easier to be nice to others and when I was nice to others I automatically felt better about myself.

Life does have a way of working in circles and what we put out we get back — eventually — but once we realize this success pattern we can see how immature it is to harm our bodies with drugs, alcohol, the wrong food and even the wrong friends. These things only deaden our feelings to the real joys in life. The happiness that might come from drugs is like an illusion we might see in a desert mirage. It isn't really there at all. But the various drugs we use don't just disappear they actually harm the body and mind causing the prime factor in aging, stress.

According to research done by the Rockefeller Foundation over 95 percent of the people born in this world are born healthy. But what makes us age and die prematurely are our own bad habits: i.e., drugs, excessive alcohol, smoking, overeating or eating the wrong foods, not enough exercise or sleep — everything that I have discussed in this book.

But just to give you a bit more research statistics, we now know at least 80 percent of the 98,000 people who die from lung cancer every year could have been saved if they had just stopped smoking. The mortality rate from heart disease is 3.6 times higher in smokers than non-smokers. I have often wondered just how much of this addiction is purely physical and how much is an unconscious dislike for ourselves.

If we cut down on our animal fat intake, do not smoke, exercise more and curb our salt intake the annual death rate from heart attacks, 638,000 yearly, would be greatly reduced.

But, we have to first like ourselves enough to maintain the self-control that enables us to take charge of our own lives. First you have to decide if you are really worth it. Many people do not consciously realize how they feel about themselves but their outer actions show it to everyone else.

If you smoke, drink too much, take drugs and eat junk, you are actually saying, "I don't like me."

The ironic part about this is that most people worry that other people won't like them when they should worry more about not liking themselves. Personally, I can cope with exterior rejection, I always rationalize by saying to myself, "Oh well, it's their loss." But I could not cope with interior rejection, that's really my loss.

Sometimes I hear a friend say, "it's too late to change even though I'm miserable I'll just have to put up with it." Nothing could be further from the truth. The old cliche is true, "It's never too late." I mean that literally. It is never too late, right up until the time when we draw our last breath on planet earth.

I once heard a marvelous story and it's worth repeating here. A very old woman was lying on her death bed with her family gathered around her. Someone in the bedside group muttered something and the old woman opened her eyes and asked, "What was that?" They were all surprised by her response and one said, "Oh, mother, it was nothing important." But she replied, "Listen, I may be dying but I'm still learning."

"ONE AND ONLY YOU"

Every single blade of grass,
And every flake of snow —
Is just a wee bit different . . .
There's no two alike, you know.

From something small, like grains of sand,
To that gigantic star
All were made with this in mind:
To be just what they are!

How foolish then, to imitate —
How useless to pretend!
Since each of us comes from a mind
Whose ideas never end.

There'll only be just one of me
To show what I can do —
And you should likewise feel quite proud
There's only one of you.

LOST LOVE

And for those who have loved and lost, the following bit of prose may help you to sustain yourself. I don't know who wrote it, but bless them.

COMES THE DAWN

"After a while you learn the subtle difference between holding a hand and chaining a soul. You learn that love doesn't mean security and you begin to learn that kisses are not contracts, presents are not promises and you begin to accept defeats with your head up and your eyes open, with the face of an adult, not the grief of a child, and you learn to build your roads on today because tomorrows ground is too uncertain and futures have a way of falling down in midflight.

After a while you learn that even sunshine burns if you get too much. So plant your own garden and decorate your own soul instead of waiting for someone to bring you flowers.

You learn that you really can endure, you really are strong, you really do have worth and you learn and learn, with every goodbye you learn."

HEIRS OF THE GODS

One last word about our immune systems. Have you ever wondered why when two people are exposed to the same disease one will get it and the other will not. This is a factor that science is not able to explain. But, obviously disease has a depressing effect on our entire body causing our mental, physical and magnetic energies to be out of balance thus in disharmony. What science has not been able to explain, religion has. Preachers readily tell us that greed and materialism cause disharmony. That's ironic, because the old saying, "You can't take it with you!" couldn't be more accurate on this planet. When we are born our biological clock starts ticking and we really only have a small amount of time here.

Still many of us think that what we profit from the most here is material goods. But actually what we profit from the most are the lessons we learn in life and the good works we manage to do. Did you ever think about how good you feel when you help someone or show kindness? Wouldn't it be a wonderful world if we could all realize that simple truth. There would be no more cruelty and hate, no more bigotry and prejudice, no more envy, jealousy and murders; and for anyone who's looking to save money we could save billions on defense because there would be no more wars.

But what makes us behave the way we do? All of us are curious about our origins and it is interesting that the controversy still rages on between Darwin's theory of evolution and the fundamentalist belief that God made us all. I have always felt that both theories might be true. Perhaps we evolved to a certain point and then God or a greater mind than ours helped to evolve us to where we are now. Science is still wondering where the missing link is.

In a book entitled; "Heirs of the Gods" by Lee and Vivianne Gladden, Ph.D.'s, there is a space age interpretation of the Bible. The Gladdens' use etymology to advance this theory. Etymology is the study of the original meaning of a word. They uncovered the root meanings of biblical passages and in their chapter, "The Experimental Creation" they state:

"Was man created outright, as the Bible claims, or did he evolve by stages shown in the fossil record? One of the most important discoveries to come out of our space age interpretation of the Bible is the answer to this question. And, curiously, the answer is both, man evolved and was then re-created by extraterrestrials.

"The Bible tells us this added agency was the activity of Celestials who refashioned him in their own other worldly image. Unfortunately, it tells us little more. How they refashioned him, their motives in doing so, the techniques they used — all these we must reconstruct from other sources. In this chapter we will attempt this reconstruction from the fragmentation hints given in the Bible and two other sources — our own emerging science of genetic engineering and paleoanthropology. The story that emerges is a truly astounding one, for it proves man is indeed "not from the apes" but is the heir of a "very different sort of ancestor."

"Normally, hundreds of thousands of years are insufficient to produce major changes in a species. Yet in the case of modern man we find a most astonishing exception to this rule. For our ancestors of only a little over 30,000 years ago lived scarcely above the level of the beasts around them. The fossil record shows they lived at this same level since they first appeared around 250,000 years ago. Suddenly, about 30,000 years ago, subtly different Homo sapiens appeared. Though their fossils look much the same as those earlier humans the quality of their intellectual functioning shows an incredible leap into the future. Humans alone, of all living creatures, aspire to the godlike condition of immortality."

The Gladdens go into great detail explaining the human family tree and I must confess that it wasn't until after I read "Heirs of the Gods" that the Bible really made sense to me. It took a space age interpretation of the Bible for the ancient literature to come to life in todays world. The Gladden's methodology was original research in this area and explained that we had evolved to a certain point when extraterrestrials which they call "Celestials" landed in a space ship somewhere around the fertile valley of the Nile. There the Celestials set up a laboratory and chose people who were living in that valley to perform genetic engineering on.

They experimented on our ancestors in order to raise their intelligence to a point comparable with their own. But, unfortunately the Celestials were sabotaged by one of their own, Satan, and therefore we still remain an unfinished experiment. This could be why scientists have never been able to come up with the missing link.

Is this why humans always seem to have problems and be in a constant state of confusion between body and mind?

What we refer to as natural are the basic body functions, the animal part of our natures. But our minds were improved far beyond our animal natures and therefore we are in constant conflict.

When we were told to increase and multiply there were very few of us on this planet. Now we have billions of humans on earth and pollution is contaminating earth, water and air. Now is the time to use

God given intelligence to plan ahead. Quality is always more desirable than quantity therefore it should be obvious that we need to limit our numbers in order to stop the nuclear and chemical pollution of our atmosphere. Our resources are not infinite they are finite and we are currently using them up at an accelerated rate thereby destroying the quality of life not only for ourselves but for our children as well.

When I explained this to my children they said it was too big a project for them to which I replied, "You can start by cleaning up your rooms!" Funny as that may sound at first, when we think about it if everyone just cleaned up their own environment we would not have pollution. We wouldn't have to worry about chemicals polluting our planet because nobody would have dumped them to begin with. All it takes to make a difference is a little more use of that great intelligence "God" gave us.

Now anyone who has lost a loved one the Neptune Society has a touching thought provoking and comforting poem.

> "Do not stand by my grave and weep
> I am not there, I do not sleep.
> I am a thousand winds that blow,
> I am the diamond glints on snow.
> I am the sun on ripened grain,
> I am the gentle autumn rain.
> When you awake in the morning's hush,
> I am the swift uplifting rush of
> Quiet birds in circled flight.
> I am the stars that shine at night.
> Do not stand by my grave and cry,
> I am not there, I did not die."

Hugh Downs wrote a list he calls the 10 myths of growing old and I'd like to reiterate them here with some side comments of my own.

- Old is a matter of age. (Nonsense: I've met old people in their 20's and young ones in their 60's.)

- You can't do anything about getting old. (Yes, you can. You can fight back in many ways, as you know, from reading this book.)

- You won't feel good when you get old. (Oh, really? I feel better now than I did 20 years ago.)

- Sex holds no interest for old people. (That depends on the old people. And has been disproven in medical studies.)

- Aging slows thinking. (Only if you let it.)

- If you're over 50, you won't make it in the work force. (You will if you look and feel good.)

- Older people should be with people their own age. (Only if they prefer people of their own age.)

- Old people are most likely to become depressed. (Not necessarily. Oddly enough, statistics show that young people are the ones most prone to suicide.)

- When you're old, you're passed your prime. (Your prime is now. Whatever your age may be.)

- You can't change people's attitudes about aging. (Well, I'm sure trying because I believe life is what you make it.)

HAPPINESS

Happiness is the great paradox in nature. It can grow in any soil, live under any condition, it defies environment. Happiness comes from within.

Happiness consists not in having, but in being. Not in possessing, but in enjoying. A martyr at the stake might have happiness that a king on a throne might envy. Woman and man are the creators of their own happiness, it is the aroma of life lived in harmony with high ideals.

Happiness is the souls joy in the possession of the intangible. It is the warm glow of a heart at peace with itself.

Only one life that soon is passed, only what's done with love will last!

Now you have my 5 point plan for delaying wrinkles. It's really not difficult to follow and certainly the rewards of a happier, healthier, better looking you are worth the effort. Only you can make this plan enjoyable and once you acquire the healthy habits they will help you become more beautiful.

Here's to Health!

ABOUT THE AUTHOR

Devra Z. Hill exemplifies the spreading belief that today's patient is tomorrow's physician.

In failing health herself several years ago, she sought help from medical doctors, but none were able to help her. She decided to take matters into her own hands, learning all she could about health and nutrition in order to regain and sustain optimum health.

She earned a Master of Science degree in nutrition from Donsbach University School of Nutrition and a Ph.D. in communications from Golden State University.

With knowledge and a daily regime of nutrition, physical exercise, meditation and her inherently cock-eyed optimist attitude she personally restored herself to good health.

Highly sought as a nutrition counselor and public speaker, Dr. Hill is the author of several books and has written for major magazines on numerous subjects. She hosts her own radio show in California and guests frequently on other radio and TV programs.

She and her husband, Hollywood publicist Irwin Zucker, are the parents of three daughters, Lori, Judi and Shari; the last two being twins and co-authors of two natural foods cookbooks.

Devra is listed in Who's Who of American Women, Foremost Women in Communications, Distinguished Authors in America and Great Britain and the International Biographical Society.

A native of San Francisco, she now resides in Beverly Hills, California. For relaxation she likes to bicycle, play tennis, jog and garden.